Tendon and Ligament Healing

TENDON AND LIGAMENT HEALING

A New Approach Through Manual Therapy

William Weintraub

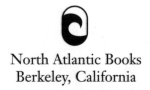

North Atlantic Books
Berkeley, California

Published by
North Atlantic Books
P.O. Box 12327
Berkeley, California 94712

Cover art by Don Jacot and Paula Koepke
Cover design by Catherine Campaigne and A/M Studios
Drawings and photographs by Don Jacot
Book design by A/M Studios
Printed in the United States of America

Tendon and Ligament Healing: A New Approach through Manual Therapy is sponsored by the Society for the Study of Native Arts and Sciences, a nonprofit educational corporation whose goals are to develop an educational and crosscultural perspective linking various scientific, social, and artistic fields; to nurture a holistic view of arts, sciences, humanities, and healing; and to publish and distribute literature on the relationship of mind, body, and nature.

LIBRARY OF CONGRESS CATALOGING-IN-PUBLICATION DATA
Weintraub, William, 1945–
   Tendon and ligament healing : a new approach through manual therapy /
William Weintraub.
   p. cm.
"Sponsored by the Society for the Study of Native Arts and Sciences"—T.p. verso.
   Includes bibliographical references.
   ISBN 1-55643-283-6
1. Tendons—Wounds and injuries—Physical therapy. 2. Ligaments—Wounds and injuries—Physical therapy. 3. Manipulation (Therapeutics) I. Society for the Study of Native Arts and Sciences. II. Title.
[DNLM: 1. Tendon injuries—rehabilitation. 2. Ligaments—Injuries. 3. Manipulation, Orthopedic. 4. Chronic Disease—rehabilitation. WE 600 W424t 1998]
RC688.W45 1999
617.4'74044—dc21
DNLM/DLC
for Library of Congress   98-17726
                                                                              CIP

1 2 3 4 5 6 7 8 9 / 03 02 01 00 99

Contents

Acknowledgments

Thanks to all my teachers, patients, and students for the development of my work. Thanks to my father, Louis Weintraub. To my overall mentor, Lew Colburn. To Neala Haze, partner through many phases. I've been fortunate to have so much help with this book: special thanks to Shierry Nicholsen for wise guidance, Don Jacot for illustrations and photos, Ayelet Maida for design, and to David Lippincott, Betsy Partridge, Paul Boudakian, Alan Leveton, Cathy Adachi, Winnie Ganshaw, and Paula Koepke.

Preface

Bill Weintraub, M.A. is at the same time an excellent therapist and a researcher who has produced a very valuable, highly interesting work in the area of tendon and ligament treatment. This book is clear and comprehensive. It is a great pleasure for me to write this preface because it is due to people like him that manual therapy gains increased acceptance in the medical world.

A therapist who is effective in relieving people's suffering deserves our encouragement and gratitude for providing help to other practitioners in the areas of treatment and research; it's so important to share our experience with others.

Modern physiology teaches us that the finest and most sensitive proprioceptors are located in tendons and ligaments. Relieving stress on the mechanoreceptors located in these structures produces specific effects through local feedback systems, permitting the release of joint and muscle problems. These nerve receptors are also part of a larger feedback loop which can provide a general benefit to the body through spinal, cerebellar, and brain stimulation. Weintraub's thorough, precise treatment methods for the tendon or ligament stimulate neural input which emanates from that local structure, and is received centrally by the organism; this causes a favorable reciprocal effect on the localized injury area from the Central Nervous System.

The structural and neural activity described above also allows beneficial repatterning of larger body functions such as orchestration of complex movements, permitting the patient to feel better in his or her life. In these ways the health of tendons and ligaments plays a role in both physical and emotional homeostasis. The soundly-based treatment options presented in this book for recovery from chronic injury bring benefits on multiple levels.

Effective treatment of these injuries is a crucial and challenging area of health care, welcoming Bill Weintraub's promising new approach here. This is why his work with osteopathic and related therapies is such an important contribution in this field.

Jean-Pierre Barral, D.O.

Preface

It gives me pleasure to write this preface to *Tendon and Ligament Healing* by Bill Weintraub. I believe this is an important publication because of the skills, light, and optimism it brings to the problem of chronic tendon/ligament injuries. The book will be helpful to anyone engaged in therapy of joints and soft tissue, especially of the tendon and ligament variety—or anyone who has sustained this type of injury and has not made satisfactory recovery. It will hold strong interest for the person who is drawn to a health care model based on the self-corrective powers of the body.

Weintraub crafted his own professional training instead of following the traditional and highly organized schools of medicine or physiotherapy, where treatment modalities are quite standardized. He escaped a certain pessimism so often inherent in the standard treatment of chronic tendon and ligament injuries. The underpinnings of his training were experiential in nature involving sports, yoga and dance. He had already embodied a sense of optimum form and function within his own body before he began his more formal study of anatomy and pathology. As he entered into the healing arts he studied with people who themselves came from personal experience and nontraditional sources. He was influenced by acupressure and Chinese theory of wholeness, and studied at length with innovative osteopaths who were continuing to expand possibilities based on deeper understanding of anatomy and touch.

With this training and background Weintraub was not limited to the traditional teachings of chronic tissue injury. He experientially learned the micro-anatomy of ligaments and tendons through touch; and he has developed a creative approach, using in-depth manual skills to aid chronic injury and dysfunction. The method is firmly grounded in osteopathic tradition. In addition, realizing the importance of the whole person, he went full circle to involve the patient in their own healing process. This book is full of useful suggestions. His combined approach has been successful and has led to an optimistic attitude for a person's recovery, which itself aids the process.

The personal application of his own methods and beliefs help validate what he presents in this book. When Weintraub sustained a chronic tendon injury from excessive weight lifting, he applied his methodology to his own injury and recovered, despite a negative prognosis given by several orthopedists. He actualized the famous axiom 'physician heal thyself.'

Bill Weintraub is to be congratulated for his insights, optimism and a fresh approach to chronic tendon and ligament problems. His understanding of how to specifically benefit the micro-anatomy through touch and his inclusion of the whole person in healing offer new possibilities for therapists and patients alike when dealing with these difficult problems. This is a timely book.

Fritz Frederick Smith, M.D.

TENDON AND LIGAMENT HEALING

CHAPTER 1

Overview

This book responds to a major challenge in the health care field. A high incidence of serious, chronic tendon and ligament injury causes substantial disability. Frequently there are unsuccessful results from the most widely used treatment. Tendons and ligaments when seriously damaged are not among the body parts more amenable to healing. I have made it a strong priority to find an effective method for reversing these injuries. The standard medical view is that nonsurgical treatment has almost no chance of success once the injury has become chronic. Surgery is in many cases only partially satisfactory or (in the long term) not so at all.

In twenty-five years of practicing structural/osteopathic manual therapy I have done considerable work with seriously damaged tendons and ligaments with some beneficial results that would be considered highly improbable by conventional medicine. I have developed a therapeutic model for treating these injuries. People in chronic cases who have exhausted the standard physiotherapy and are facing surgery can have a viable option for recovery, which is thoroughly described in this book.

Through a view of my innovative treatment approach and recent scientific research findings the book explores the active function and treatment of an often overlooked area (tendons and ligaments). This brings to light a basic bodily healing response, which can be important for strong self-maintenance and tissue healing of any part of the body. The story of the dancer Julia L., on the next page, is a capsule picture of strategy to promote this process. The research points to primary yet little-known properties of tendons/ligaments that have highly favorable implications for their recovery potential.

The book's focus on manual therapy for ligament and tendon injury illustrates possibilities beyond the standard medical model for a creative approach to health care based on the body as a dynamic, responsive organism. Adaptability of the body is one of the essential principles, emerging from my clinical work and long-term exploration of health and physical awareness.

Clear, active perception is a key skill I use as a clinician. My therapy model combines this with well-trained technical/anatomical precision to apply its manual techniques for the body structure. Two in-depth case accounts and ten capsule case reports in Chapter 4 directly illustrate this approach, along with the following brief account featuring the obstacles and therapy process of a chronic tendon injury.

Julia L. is a lifelong dancer who was very discouraged when she initially consulted me for a persistent problem with her right knee. A tall woman of forty-two and now cochair of a university dance department, she had stopped her workouts and was unable to demonstrate for her classes. Fifteen months earlier, when starting to dance after prolonged sitting on the floor of a cold studio, she noticed pain and stiffness of her posterior, lateral knee that became a constant ache and burning sensation. This had continued and worsened despite various medications, physiotherapy, chiropractic, and periods of rest. She was unable to bend her knee with any weight-bearing without weakness and a lot of pain. She was quite disconsolate as she had been forced to reduce her teaching schedule and worried about her future in the profession to which she was very devoted.

An MRI scan revealed a substantial tear of the biceps femoris (lateral hamstring) tendon behind the knee joint. Four months after the initial injury two orthopedic surgeons felt there was no longer a realistic hope of recovery with conservative care. They proposed surgical repair of the tendon, which Julia was reluctant to undergo.

Julia agreed to my initial suggestion of three weekly treatments to see if the structural/osteopathic therapy I practice could help her injury. I found significant swelling of her posterior knee, along with adhesion, weakness, "stringiness," and a twisted alignment pattern of the tendon fibers as well as a palpable divot in the tendon where it had been torn. I used gentle techniques to specifically free, align, and tone the tendon fibers, as well as free restrictions of her lower spine and lower abdominal viscera. Julia was cooperative in maintaining reduced activity levels and a moderate exercise program. We both noticed that gradually her range and ease of knee joint mobility was increasing, swelling and inflammation was reduced, and pain was subsiding.

After four weeks the frequency of treatments was reduced to two- and then

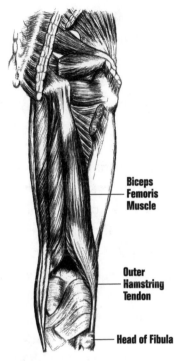

Biceps Femoris Muscle

Outer Hamstring Tendon

Head of Fibula

FIGURE 1
Posterior view of right biceps femoris (lateral hamstring) muscle and its tendon at the knee.

three-week intervals. I continued to treat restrictions of her calf muscles and fascias, damage to the neighboring popliteal tendon, and a stubborn fixation of the ankle joint and cuboid bone in her right foot. After ten weeks she could climb a flight of stairs without pain and comfortably walk one mile with moderate hills. She was optimistic enough to be choreographing a piece in which she hoped to dance. With continued manual therapy techniques the tendon fibers had been realigned, their tone strengthened, adhesions almost eliminated, and the defect in the tendon was filling in well.

At sessions three and then five months from starting therapy Julia could extend her knee completely and flex it to 110 degrees and then 135 degrees comfortably with weight-bearing (within 5 degrees of normal). She was demonstrating for her classes with progressive ease and increasing her workouts. I found that the torn part of the tendon was very close to being intact and that the texture of the whole tendon was more resilient, "bouncy," with almost no laxity. Treatments went to one-month intervals, and after four of these Julia received two orthopedic evaluations of her knee as being normal. At that time she was very relieved and happy to resume a full teaching and workout schedule. She continued to feel quite well the following year.

Julia's story is very hopeful considering the extent and duration of her tendon injury. Hers was one of the high proportion of seriously damaged tendons and ligaments that become chronic. She had availed herself of the standard medical (and some nonmedical) treatments with the exception of surgery, about which she was hesitant in part because of uncertainty about its outcome. Julia had no major health problems preventing recovery and was quite cooperative through the course of treatment; these are important factors for the success of my therapy in the case of a stubborn condition.

This account portrays strategies that reflect basic principles of structural health care, which have become clear through years in this field. These include the importance of precise anatomical focus and capacity to work with subtle changes of structure. Another essential principle is illustrated by my combining detailed, specific treatment of the small fibers and tissues of the local injury area with an overall approach to improving larger body patterns and tensions. Therapeutic techniques for Julia's spine, muscles, fascias, visceral structures, and other joints helped to normalize the forces connected to the injury zone and promote its recovery. Progression of her case emphasizes the basic principle of responsiveness and self-corrective capacity of body tissues when given proper conditions. Focus on this capacity will allow insight into various elements of body function.

Including its elements that are instructional for therapists, the book's primary theme is an informational source and guide that is both useful and provocative. This can shed light on the role of the therapist, self-help with injury, and sports/movement training. It addresses the question of what are realistic expectations for the function, health, and in-depth treatment of ligaments and tendons?

A Manual Therapy Model—A New Approach

The primary techniques I used in Julia's case (and in all of my practice) are the osteopathic methods of Strain-Counterstrain, cranial and visceral osteopathy, and Fascial Release, as well as Body-Mind Centering. Also utilized are techniques from Zero Balancing, and from acupressure therapy, which was my initial training and licensing. All of these methods individually and sometimes in combination have valuable aspects for treatment of tendons/ligaments, which will be discussed in later sections. I first worked with large numbers of these injuries in the mid-1970s when much of my practice in New York City consisted of dancers. Since then it has been a full-time practice involving all the major areas of structural health. These include: lower back and other spinal problems in the cervical area, visceral restrictions, nerve impingements, the cranial area, and peripheral joints (shoulder, ankle, etc.).

What actual changes occur in the ligament or tendon tissue during the healing process? Some are seen in Julia's recovery (e.g. reduction of adhesions) and there are a number of others that will be illustrated. What is changed in the interaction of that tissue with surrounding structures, fluids, and neural function? There is not much available literature with well-woven description of structural and functional events that are vital in tendon/ligament recovery. The book relates these physical shifts of recovery to the therapy method(s) I use to promote the change.

The role of manual therapy in the conventional health care system is still very limited. In a system involving steep costs for highly technological and hospital-based interventions, incorporating the option of a noninvasive, effective treatment could be attractive.

My manual therapy model for treating these injuries consists of:

1. The osteopathic and other structural therapies that have been mentioned.

2. The way that I combine these methods and the specific usages to which they are directed.

3. The skills and aptitudes necessary for effective application of the techniques. This includes certain perceptual skills and thorough knowledge of anatomy and kinesiology.

This model I've developed represents a new approach to serious, chronic tendon and ligament injuries for a number of reasons:

- In the standard medical system in which most patients in this society are treated, manual therapy in any form is not an accepted strategy for reversing and healing significant damage to tendons/ligaments once their condition has become chronic. While some physiotherapists train beyond the standard approach, conventional theory and practice is definite that surgery is the only method with a realistic chance of success in this situation.

- Most of the therapy techniques in the model are innovative and not well known, and I have thorough technical training in them.

- Application of these techniques is done in some original ways.

- The means by which the methods are combined is uncommon.

- Certain skills and aptitudes used to apply the clinical techniques (e.g. fine perception to detect subtle changes of structure and larger body patterns) are unusual; this is particularly the case in relation to applying these abilities to systematic, structurally accurate treatment of tendons and ligaments.

- There is a level of very specific, anatomically precise, in-depth manual work with the often fragile intricacies of the ligament or tendon microstructure, and the methods are inventive. These include particular strategies I use for aligning the small tendon fibers and their bundles, restoring their tone and reversing laxity, and working with the electrical activity of the tissues.

These features of my therapeutic model indicate its new approach for this type of injury. It is not expected that clinicians utilize every element of the model, but that all will find important areas for exploration and focus.

Certain factors are positive or negative indicators for potential success in the application of my therapy in cases of serious injury. To present the positive side here, an important favorable indicator is the patient's cooperation with recommendations for exercise and for reduced activity to avoid aggravation. Julia L., whose tendon treatment was mentioned earlier, is a good example of this. Also helpful are adequate nutrition and general health including absence of systemic disturbance of the connective tissue. The presence of certain negative factors (e.g. continued overuse or a connective tissue disorder) would greatly reduce the likelihood of full recovery. When the injury is severe it is vital for a successful outcome that the patient wants to recover.

There are possible benefits in skilled movement and postural therapy, nutritional therapy including dietary supplements, and strategies for stress reduction. All these can be beneficial for tendon/ligament injury and can be useful in combination with my manual treatment. An example of this is that in many cases I find it quite important to help the subjects improve the efficiency of their movement patterns (including occupational usage) to avoid further injury.

In addition, there are many other methods besides these three by which tendons and ligaments are treated in both standard and complementary medicine. While many have some positive effect they are often limited in treating the serious, chronic injuries that are the focus of this book. These conditions generally do not reach a positive outcome with most therapies. I will not examine all of the methods here, but it will be important to discuss the standard medical treatment because it is received by most patients in this society. That discussion provides a clear reference point for viewing my approach.

The central topic of this book is presented in part as a research study determining the effectiveness of my therapy model for chronic injury. Case studies from my clinical work will be used as a primary example, and related to scientific findings and theories. This helps to provide a clear overall vision of the book's variety of material.

Sequence of the Book

Main features of the book are linked here to its progression.

The nature of tendons and ligaments is described in Chapter 2. I feel this presents important insights into physiological processes of healing in these structures. Portrayal of their composition and function is basic for looking into injury and recovery mechanisms. These are a foundation for the case studies and the entire topic. Primary information about these connective tissue structures begins Chapter 2 and will lead to the conventional medical perspective on their function and healing capacity. This is followed by recent scientific research findings and theory that alter and expand this widely accepted outlook.

In the standard model ligaments and tendons are relatively passive. Recent information and outlook demonstrates a more active, vital function. There is a general sense of the dynamism of body tissues. Creative concepts of tendons/ligaments are originated by such researcher/clinicians as Bainbridge Cohen, Korr, F. Smith, R. Becker, Hunt, and Studitskii. Their theories amplify scientific research findings on the health aspects of connective tissue neural involvement, electro-magnetic activity, cellular function, and its process of tissue regeneration. Ideas for effective manual therapy methods and other health-enhancing strategies clearly emerge from this material.

In Chapter 3, "A Manual Therapy Model for Tendon and Ligament Injury," I describe my therapeutic approach. This includes a view of the various techniques and the skills and aptitudes needed to apply them effectively. The chapter opens with an outline of the standard medical treatment for tendon and ligament injury that is so widely utilized in this society. Its prevalence makes it an important reference point for viewing my working strategy.

There is an overview of each of the principle techniques in the model and explanation of how I use it to address an injured tendon or ligament. Certain essential principles are common to the techniques and these are listed later in the chapter. Another section compares my approach for these injuries to that of the standard model. In dramatizing the central points and overall scheme of the two strategies this comparison furnishes a perspective on both, and on conservative care in general. I feel this will be a practical clarification of important factors for clinical success with difficult injury cases.

The techniques section presents main features and fine points of the techniques, and usages that are both regular and unorthodox. While it has many instructional elements and can be useful to clinicians in a number of ways, it is not primarily a training manual. It will be informative as to why and how a method is employed and where it is particularly beneficial (especially in regard to tendon/ligament injury). Although this does not preclude what I regard as the necessity of learning one or more of the techniques very thoroughly, there is illustration of how techniques in combination can be utilized effectively for injury cases. Portrayal of the individual elements (techniques, etc.) and their interweaving into an overall approach that makes up this model may afford readers from various backgrounds a sense that can also be applied to a range of structural (and other) health issues.

A vital element of my working strategy is the abilities and aptitudes that are used to apply the manual techniques. My route to learning these skills and techniques is chronicled in a discussion of personal background and training. The account provides some illustration of how and why the model has been developed in this form. It shows how interests and experience have been an influence in my professional training and in the application of the techniques. One major influence is my own recovery from a serious tendon injury.

The two case study presentations in Chapter 4 are thorough accounts of the course of therapy for a serious, chronic tendon injury and a corresponding ligament injury. These are information-rich cases selected for study in depth. They are examples of essential aspects of tendons and ligaments and my usage of the manual methods. After each account there is a case-progression chart tracing a sequence of variables over the course of therapy. Ten shorter case accounts form the chapter's last section, adding breadth and showing a variety of situations for using this approach.

The main variables traced in the cases are 1) comfort/pain, 2) range of motion, 3) level of function, and 4) clinical findings such as tissue quality of the tendon/ligament. These are central to in the book's research study which evaluates therapeutic efficacy of my approach, with conclusions drawn in Chapter 7. The beginning of the fourth chapter describes the case-study research methodology I am using, which is very useful in real-life situations (e.g., events in a clinical practice). This provides a perspective on the case accounts which are the main part of the chapter.

Chapter 5 describes the processes and tissue changes as a tendon or ligament recovers from chronic injury. It is timely to see a systematic viewing of functional and anatomical changes important in their healing process. There is not much detail in the available literature. Also notable is the look at how each of these changes can be promoted by methods from the therapy model; this allows a more fully textured sense of the recovery process related to a conservative care (nonsurgical) method.

In Chapter 6 I present self-help strategies for chronic ligament or tendon injuries. While this is not a substitute for professional treatment of serious injuries, it can be a useful adjunct. There are ideas for when and where people can seek treatment and other practical means of aiding your own progress.

Chapter 7 is an overview and a discussion of the case studies. It relates these accounts to primary topics such as healing capacity of tendons/ligaments and vital changes for recovery. The cases are seen in light of various aspects of my therapy model. There is also a section of further thoughts on important tools for a practitioner to effect positive results with serious injuries. These skills involve a central role of the therapist as instrument.

Chapter 7 presents conclusions and an overview related to the possibilities raised in the book for:

- a more potent healing response of ligaments and tendons,

- a fresh view of health care principles in a new approach to chronic injury, and

- benefits of manual therapy.

My central focus in the book is a grounding in information on the above topics, leading to a sense of greater possibility.

CHAPTER 2

The Nature of Tendons and Ligaments

Preview

A range of information in this chapter provides insight for the entire topic. I have selected material on tendons/ligaments that is vital for understanding their recovery from injury and the therapy I am using. The story of the dancer, Julia L., in Chapter 1 refers to my work with adhesions and laxity of her injured tendon and the alignment pattern of its fibers—and a steady recovery process. These structural and metabolic features are given an informational basis in this chapter.

The material here reveals much promise for the potential of these connective tissues to heal. The account starts with basic structure and function. Following are standard medical views and then the perspective of innovative theory and research. This introductory preview and a chapter summary will acquaint less technically-oriented readers with the essentials of the material.

Grounding in the basic structure begins with a view of collagen fibers, fibroblasts, and ground substance (building blocks of tendons and ligaments). This proceeds to their essential properties such as viscoelasticity and tensile strength. The passive structures seen in the conventional model do not inherently produce movement; when stretched past a certain point the tissue cannot regain its normal resting length and will remain lax. When the process of injury becomes serious it results in major tearing of fibers, adhesions, and loss of function. Portrayal of the central, primary mechanisms of inflammation and chronic injury syndrome may inform us as to how they can be reversed.

Following is a section in which I describe findings from recent scientific research enriching the standard perspective. Intriguing clues in this material lead to avenues through which manual therapy can benefit the injured structures. Normal connective tissue (e.g., tendons and ligaments) continuously remodels itself for regular healthy maintenance. There is increasing evidence that these tissues are equipped to repair themselves from injury by manufacturing large amounts of collagen and ground substance.

Through new information the traditionally held view of the neural function of ligaments is expanded to a more active one; they are involved in complex neuromuscular feedback circuits. Data indicates that the richly innervated, responsive tendons/ligaments play a substantial role in neural control of movement and posture. Research in electromagnetism points to its important bodily influence on internal reporting of and response to injury, along with reparative growth. Connective tissue appears to react readily to this form of energy, which is also linked to the acupuncture system. This has intriguing implications for its healing potential and for treatment strategies, as does research on the properties of cells.

Studies in cell biology yield evidence for contractile capacity of nonmuscle cells, including the fibroblasts of tendon and ligament tissue. Cellular contraction and capacity for locomotion indicates strong possibilities of the tissue to generate forces from within itself. Those activities could increase its tone when it is weak and also assist reversal of laxity; this lengthened condition of chronically overstretched ligaments is usually thought to be irreversible without invasive procedures.

Other potentially valuable cellular aspects of connective tissue health are found in research on satellite (stem) cells. These relatively simple cells are active in regeneration of damaged muscle. A cellular cycle of despecialization into stem cells leading to their respecialization in order to form healthy tissue may be operative for injury reversal in all body tissues. The conditions that promote regeneration are described as the "plastic state." This state is a component of a basic bodily healing response, which I describe in the summary at the end of the chapter.

This chapter is a backdrop for the cases of the people reported in Chapter 4, and defines the whole topic. The latter part of the material here includes the insightful theories of some pioneering researcher/clinicians in the field. Their views on tendons/ligaments round out the chapter's picture of relatively dynamic, interactive structures. From my standpoint, there is some fascination with the scientific evidence of vitality and sophistication embodied in these tissues.

Structure, Composition

Tendons and ligaments are dense, regular connective tissue structures (bands, cords, or straps) with mostly parallel fiber arrangement. Connective tissue has much variety, but in general it is characterized by the presence of a large extracellular matrix and a wide dispersion of cells.[1, 2] The *cellular* portion of tendons and ligaments are the fibroblasts that synthesize and maintain the fibers and the ground substance.

The *extracellular* matrix consists of ground substance and fibers. The ground substance is the nonfibrous component of the matrix and is made up of glycosaminoglycans and proteoglycans. These long-chain molecules are linked to the collagen fibers to help form connective tissue. The ground substance facilitates tissue metabolism and provides support, shock absorption, and resiliency. It also decreases friction and attracts and binds water. Water occupies the largest percentage of weight (and space) in all tissues (60 to 80 percent).[3] The varying percentage of water-binding protein contained in the ground substance affects the hydration level of the tissue.

The fibrous component of the matrix is primarily collagen fibers, with some elastin. This is the support framework and comprises 75 to 80 percent of the dry weight of tendons and ligaments. Collagen is the most abundant protein in the human body; its basic building blocks are amino acids, primarily proline, glycine, and lysine. Its amino acid chains assemble into long triple helix molecules by hydrogen bonding to oxygen radicals along the chains. The molecules line up side-by-side to attach by intermolecular bonding, which forms the hollow collagen fibers. These fibers are the individual units that also attach by molecular bonding to form bundles that comprise the overall structure of the tendon or ligament.[4, 5]

Collagen fibers have a tensile strength approaching that of steel. The parallel arrangement of the fibers is somewhat wavy in the relaxed state, and straight when under a tension pull. Dense connective tissue has more collagen fibers and less ground substance than other connective tissue. Elastin is an extensible substance that forms a small component of tendons and most ligaments. A low percentage of specialized ligaments contains a large component of elastin, which gives them increased extensibility.

Tendons and ligaments are surrounded by a sheath (called a paratenon, and unnamed for ligaments) of loose areolar connective tissue, which facilitates gliding on contiguous structures. In locations

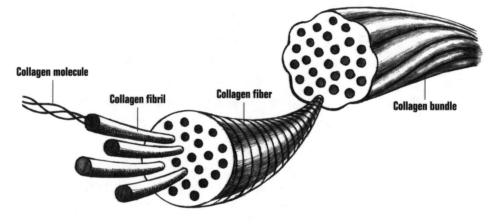

FIGURE 2
Collagen structures in tendon or ligament.

involving high-friction forces, particularly in the wrist and hand, tendons are surrounded by an additional sheath beneath the more fibrous paratenon. This is the epitenon and is a synovial tissue layer that produces synovial fluid for lubrication.[1, 6] Tendon tissue blends with muscle at one end, and at the other (similar to both ends of a ligament)

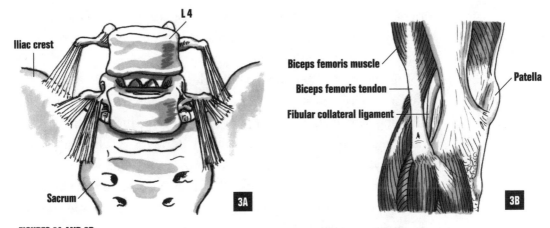

FIGURES 3A AND 3B
Ligaments and tendons in location. The iliolumbar ligaments (3A) contribute to stability of the lumbosacral area. Therapy for a biceps femoris tendon (3B) winjury (Julia L.) was described in Chapter 1.

meets with its bony attachment by blending through the fibrocartilage covering, and then into the cortical bone itself.[7] The musculotendinous junction and tendon-bone, ligament-bone junctions are often the location of injury. Ligaments are extra-capsular, intra-capsular, or are thickenings of the joint capsule. Both structures are richly innervated and have relatively little direct blood supply.

Properties, Function

The following description of the properties and function of tendons/ligaments represents the accepted view in standard medical theory. Some aspects of this view are altered in the perspective of recent theory and research. Ligaments are described as passive structures whose main function is to stabilize joints, guide their movement, and prevent excessive joint motion.[7] Tendons are also described in the standard literature as passive structures. Their main function is to transmit forces from muscle to bone and fascia.

Collagen structures are described as anisotropic, as they don't have equal mechanical properties when loaded in different directions. They exhibit properties (strength and elasticity) that vary according to their orientation in space when a constant force is applied.[1, 8] Due to their parallel fiber arrangement, tendons and ligaments are particularly adapted to resist tensile loads.

Ligaments and tendons exhibit the property of viscoelasticity. Similar to purely elastic materials, they can regain their original shape following deformation, after removal of the deforming load. When an elastic material is stretched it has work done on it, which increases its energy. It stores this energy and keeps it available, which enables the material to recoil back to its original shape. Due to the additional presence of viscosity, viscoelastic materials exhibit time-dependent properties of recoverability. Connective tissues also are temperature sensitive, which affects their rate of creep (slow elongation). To most effectively stretch out (elongate) this tissue, it should be heated and subjected to a large load over a long time period, to produce creep.[1, 6, 7]

When tendons or ligaments are subjected to sudden, prolonged, or excessive forces, the elastic limits of the tissue may be exceeded and the tissue enters the plastic range. In the plastic range the tissue is permanently deformed and is no longer able to return to its original state following removal of the deforming force. Ligaments or tendons that are thought to be incapable of returning to their original length after elongation are described as lax, or permanently elongated.[1, 7] After the plastic range is exceeded, with continued loading, the structure reaches the point of failure as the fibers rupture.

The term "load" refers to an external force applied to a structure. Two main factors determine the strength response of a ligament or tendon under loading: their size and shape, and the speed of loading. The greater the number of fibers that are oriented in the direction of loading, and the wider and thicker those fibers are, the stronger the ligament or tendon. These structures exhibit increased strength and stiffness (resistance to movement) with an increased speed of loading.[1, 7, 8]

Tendons and most ligaments have a fairly balanced combination of brittleness (resistance to force without having a plastic range) and ductility (capacity for deformation without failure). They have some brittleness and some ductility. Differing values for failure point are given in many references, but Frankel's and Adams' figures are fairly standard when they state that collagen fiber bundles reach a failure point after exceeding an elongation of either 6 to 8 percent,[7] or 10 to 15 percent.[9] This is typical for tissue with a very high percentage of parallel collagen fibers (tendons and most ligaments). Tendons and ligaments have a high degree of resilience—the capacity to absorb and store energy within the elastic range, and then readily return to the original dimension and release that energy.[5] Their normal response to intermittent tension (application and release of a tensile force) that is not excessive is an increase in thickness and strength.[1]

Connective tissue ground substance can vary from a watery sol-state to a viscous gel-state. It has the characteristic of becoming more fluid when it is stirred up, and more of a solid gel when it is colder and sits without being disturbed. With a higher metabolic rate, motion, and warmth, the energy level of the tissue is raised and the ground substance is more fluid and ductile. With a lower energy level from reduced metabolism, lower temperature, and inactivity, the ground substance is more of a gel and the tissue is less able to soften and stretch.[5]

When tendons and ligaments are subjected to prolonged immobilization they show disorganization of their parallel fiber arrangement and a decrease in their water and proteoglycan content.[3, 7, 10] The tendon or ligament insertion into the bone becomes weakened due to osteoclastic activity destroying their fibers. In some tests, ligaments that had been immobilized for eight weeks showed decreases in strength and measurements of load-to-failure of 35 to 40 percent.[3, 10, 11]

Standard Medical View of Properties, Capacity for Healing

The standard medical model of the properties and healing capacity of ligaments and tendons is that which is most prevalent for orthopedists, sports medicine physicians, and many physical therapists. In this perspective these structures are seen as *passive* structures that don't inherently produce movement. Their tension is dependent on their length. Ligaments are described as "fixed-length stays."[5, 6, 7, 12]

Viscoelastic properties are recognized, and when stretched so that their deformation is increased to the point of failure they will not be able to return to their original dimension (length). There is little or no discussion of any other property that would reverse this laxity. Paris states that overstretched ligaments can't regain tone, making it difficult to correct poor posture.[13] Subotnick's view is that fibroblasts of adult tendons are inactive, so that healing is dependent on metaplasia of surrounding fat cells.[14] The standard view is that once an injury is chronic, laxity cannot be counteracted by conservative care and can only be reversed surgically.

A characteristic opinion is expressed by the surgeon who states that "once a ligament is torn it is never going to come back all the way" (even with surgery).[15] Ligamentous fiber rupture is seen as difficult to heal, and is usually treated by surgery. Likewise for a tendon, the greater the extent to which it is torn, the higher the probability that surgery will be recommended.[6, 7, 8, 13, 14, 15] The medical perspective is that if tendinitis becomes chronic, the tendon gives way to scar and degenerative tissue and can require surgery to clean out the area. Partial rupture of the Achilles tendon will most often need surgical repair. Seeking to downplay unrealistic expectations of the possible results of surgery, Garrick states that "there are injuries that just don't get better" (even with surgery).[15] There are variations as to when an injury is defined as chronic. The orthopedist Keene defines a chronic tendon injury as one with over six to eight weeks' duration.[8] Definitions of chronic injury extend to being over six months' duration, with three or four months as fairly common.

The standard medical view of tendons and ligaments and their injuries determines their treatment in most instances. The clients in my case studies had exhausted the standard care options and had then chosen not to undergo surgery.

Neural Involvement: Standard View and Recent Research Findings

The traditional view of the innervation and resultant function of tendons and ligaments has been altered by information from some research findings since the 1960s. Ligaments are intimately related structurally with the joint capsules and have similar neural receptors. In most of the cutaneous sense organs and joint areas, the receptors are specialized, histologically modified ends of sensory nerve fibers.[2] They convert energy into action potentials. The four cutaneous senses are touch-pressure, cold, warmth, and pain. Traditionally, the receptors identified by anatomists in joint areas are the Ruffini, Pacinian, Meissner's, Merkel's, and more recently, free nerve endings. All of these are mechanoreceptors that respond to tactile stimuli. The tendons contain receptors known as Golgi tendon organs, which have close correlates found in ligaments.[2]

The traditional view was that ligaments had some of the same receptors contained in joints, and that these articular receptors function to provide some proprioception (sense of body position in space) and a protective role of supplying signals in a reflex loop with neighboring muscles. When the ligament or joint reaches the end-point of movement range it reports through paths to the spine, which in turn effect muscle contraction through stimulating the alpha motoneurons in the muscle—thereby providing a splinting action preventing further joint movement.

Recent research findings lead to a new perspective. Ligaments and joint receptors are now also seen as part of a more complex neuromuscular control system, which also operates through the smaller gamma motoneurons, located in neuromuscular spindles (stretch receptors) embedded in muscles. When the gamma neurons receive appropriate signals related to position and movement range and rate, they effect contraction of the muscle that they supply. The gamma loop is a length-regulating reflex mechanism for each muscle that is protective against excessive stretch; it is important for production of accurate, well-coordinated movement and postural control. Its functions have been brought to light relatively recently. Ligament and joint receptor signals have considerable effects on this feedback system.[16, 17, 18, 19] They affect it throughout the entire range of joint motion, and include rate of movement as another reporting variable in addition to position.[16, 19, 20]

Swedish neurophysiologists Johannsen and Sjolander report on research findings showing that joint and (particularly) ligament receptors are able to report joint angle throughout the full range of movement.[20] The presence of mid-range receptors expands on the older model that restricted signaling to the end-points of range, and shows that articular receptors contribute more substantially to movement and position sense than was previously recognized. It has also been shown recently that the complexity and diversity of articular receptors are equal to that of cutaneous receptors.[17] In addition, there is now strong evidence of rich innervation of ligaments with the same nerve types as those in joint cap-

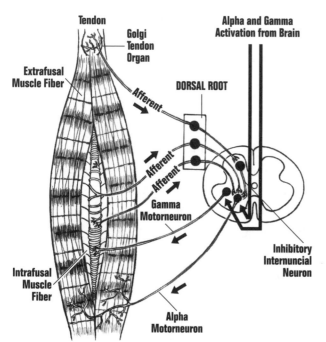

FIGURE 4
Muscle spindle and gamma neuromuscular loop. This illustrates the scheme of the gamma nerve fibers supplying the intrafusal fibers of the muscle spindle, alpha nerve fibers to the main (extrafusal) body of the muscle, and their connection with the central nervous system. The drawing indicates the influence of muscle spindle activity on the main muscle fibers.

sules, to provide varied receptor flows through the whole range of joint movement.

Nerves are now seen to fulfill an important trophic function of providing delivery of nutrients to peripheral structures such as tendons and ligaments. Korr and other investigators have elaborated this mechanism. Neurotrophic activity, the delivery of proteins by axoplasmic flow from the nerve cell body along the axon to its target tissue (both antegrade and retrograde), varies in the rate of flow and quality of the axoplasm.[16, 39] It can be compromised by structural pressures in the nerve root, along the course of the axon, and in the target tissue; it has major effects on the health of tendons and ligaments, which are so richly innervated.[16, 54] Freedom from excessive structural pressures is necessary for optimal trophic function.

These recent research findings indicate an expanded neural role for ligaments and tendons. Ligament and tendon receptors function to assist smooth coordination of movement and muscular contraction for stability, as well as contributing to position and equilibrium maintenance through signaling to the brainstem and supplying higher centers with input related to more conscious body-image.[21] Much of the nerve control of posture is located in tendons and ligaments.[17, 19] In many ways they are highly sensitive structures that play a more important neural role than is portrayed in the traditional view. This role is more responsive and complex.

Injury Process and Result, Tissue Changes

Depiction here of injury and inflammation primarily has conventional acceptance although some of the information is recent (Korr, Simkin, Radin, Viidik). It is a foundation for expansion and alteration of the standard view that resumes in the section on tissue re-modeling, through the end of the chapter.

There are some common features and characteristics of the process and result of most tendon and ligament injuries. Injuries are most likely to result from a sudden trauma, or to be more gradual and then be classified as some type of overuse injury. There are also systemically caused injuries from disease such as rheumatoid arthritis or diabetes, endocrine disorders, or from infection.[7] A tendon injury is termed tendinitis, a ligament injury usually called a sprain. Inflammation occurs, causing abnormal and impaired function of the tendon or ligament. There is some degree of rupture to the fibers of the structure, and some swelling. Tendinitis can often involve damage to the tendon sheath.

Establishing a diagnosis includes examination for instability of the joint where the tendon or ligament is located, and examination for loss of function.[8] Radiographic findings can be utilized. Injuries are often classified into three grades reflecting degree of rupture and instability.[6, 7, 8] In Grade 1 injury the ligament recovers its resting length after trauma and sustains microfailure of some fibers. In Grade 2 the structure doesn't completely recover its length, and there is some instability and a greater degree of fiber rupture. In the Grade 3 injury the tendon or ligament has a region of gross disruption of its fibers, and considerable instability. The serious injury thus consists of significant fiber tearing and loss of function.

Traumatic injury to a tendon occurs when there is sudden unanticipated stretching of an already contracted muscle, resulting in a tear of its tendon. Likewise, an unanticipated force applied to a ligament incapacitates its afferent signaling to limit joint motion via muscle antagonist contraction. Thus, the joint may undergo a substantial, sudden movement and the ligament (that is adjacent to it) can rupture.[22]

Gradual onset (overuse) tendinitis is caused when microfailure of fibers occurs from excessive repetitive loads on a tendon, or when the rest period in between loads is inadequate to enable the tendon fibers to regain their resting length. Predisposing influences are temperature extremes, excessive vibration, repetitive tasks, or usage in unusual postures.[6] Tendinitis (or ligament sprain) often starts as minute single-fiber tears. When the fibers tear they also swell. This causes them to rub against the tendon sheath, which becomes irritated and can also swell. The capacity for tendon gliding in the sheath is reduced as more and more adhesions are formed. Progression of the problem will result in a greater degree of tearing. It is common to find nodules and marked thickening in the ligament, along with a chronic low-grade inflammatory process[4] (see Figure 5, "Main Elements of tendon/ligament injury").

Inflammation in the Injury Process

Inflammation is an important aspect of tendon or ligament injury. It is a term used for a large group of normal processes provoked by damage or alien material.[2, 23] Inflammation is a bodily response to injurious agents in order to remove toxic or foreign material. It involves the infiltration of a region with white cells and extra fluid.[24, 25, 26] One part of the secondary stage of the inflammation process (starting three to five days after injury) is ingrowth of capillary buds and the appearance of fibroblasts that start to manufacture collagen and ground substance. The late stage of inflammation (as part of repair) involves the maturation and remodeling of the young connective tissue, which includes the chemical cross-linking between collagen fibers.[23, 26]

When the inflammatory process is prolonged, it causes problems for the ligament or tendon that is healing.[26] In the middle and late stage of inflammation, when there is not adequate, appropriate stress of movement for the injured structure, the developing fiber orientation will be random (not parallel). There will be excessive cross-linking of fibers resulting in the formation of dense, inflexible tissue.[23]

When lymphatic drainage is inadequate the continued edema from excess fluid results in decreased circulation from excess pressure. Edema in the joint area disrupts alignment and contact of the bone surfaces that leads to joint instability and consequent increase of ligamentous laxity. The rheumatologist Simkin reports that continued joint inflammation can compromise the capacity for lymphatic drainage, which further compounds the problem of instability.[24, 27] False strain reflexes caused by long-term inflammation result from excessive afferent nerve input to the CNS. The excessive input is partially caused by musculoskeletal tension imbalances, and also acts to maintain them (see section on neural involvement).[28] When a region remains swollen the structures are bathed in serofibrinous exudate. Fibrin, a protein needed in blood clotting, is deposited between tissue layers in tendons and ligaments, and between them and surrounding structures such as sheaths. The fibrin seals these structures in a shorter, less mobile, adhered condition.[2, 29]

The purpose of post-injury vascular events as part of the inflammatory process is to mobilize and transport the defense components of the blood (leukocytes) to the injury area, and to secure their passage through the vessel walls into the tissue spaces. When this post-injury defense mode is prolonged excessively, it interferes with the normal healing process of the tissue. A self-perpetuating cycle of irritation and inflammatory response leading to further irritation becomes a component of the chronic injury pattern.

Chronic Injury

In chronic tendon and ligament injury, the normal healing process of connective tissue is disrupted. Normal tissue remodeling is prevented by stresses (such as prolonged inflammation, inactivity) and hypovascularity.[8, 10, 25, 26] Connective tissue tends to become shorter and denser as it heals, unless it has beneficial conditions.[30] This contracture and thickening partially results from the increased interfiber bonding in a shortened state. The individual fibers lose gliding capacity and mobility relative to each other as do bundles of fibers, and whole tendons and ligaments relative to their surrounding structures (joints, capsules, sheaths). The adhesion process of fibers and layers of tissue leads to reduced extensibility and mobility.[1, 5] With poor circulation, hypoxia, and continued tearing, tissue regrowth takes the form of scar tissue as tears coalesce in portions of the ligament.[10, 26] Scar tissue is weaker than the normal type. The water content and amount of ground substance (proteoglycan content) of the tissue is reduced; there is a

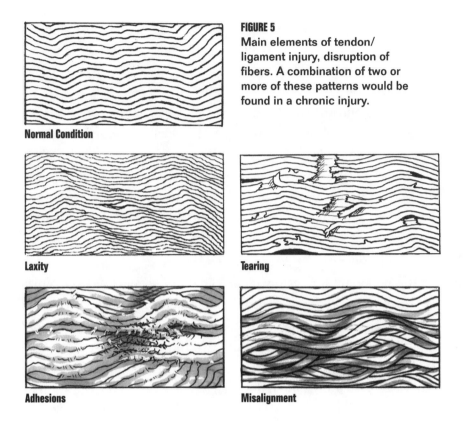

FIGURE 5
Main elements of tendon/
ligament injury, disruption of
fibers. A combination of two or
more of these patterns would be
found in a chronic injury.

Normal Condition

Laxity

Tearing

Adhesions

Misalignment

lessening of its normal ratio of ground substance to collagen fibers, which is another factor causing a denser, less pliant structural situation and impaired metabolism of the tissue.

In chronic injury the normal parallel fiber arrangement is disorganized, which reduces extensibility and strength. Prolonged low-grade inflammation is maintained along with improper lymphatic and vascular flow. This also causes abnormal metabolic function in the tissue.[8, 26] Ligaments and tendons can exhibit both hypo- and hyper-mobility. Often, both of these conditions exist in different portions of the same structure. There is a disruption of balanced neural activity, as the tendon and ligament receptors report inappropriate strain signals caused by the irritation of the tissue.[16, 31] This sets up an ongoing stress on the ligament due to muscular tension, uncoordinated movement, and joint instability; all of these factors contribute to general neurotrophic disturbance and impairment of circulation in the tissues.[16, 20, 31]

Remodeling Process of Connective Tissue

In normal, nonpathologic functioning all connective tissue is capable of healthy remodeling. Rolf asserts that it is in a continuous state of structural reorganization.[30] This self-renovation is exemplified by the response of tendons or ligaments to increased stress levels. Tissues respond to fatigue stresses (such as athletic training) by increasing the rate of tissue production (collagen fibers, ground substance). When there is proper vascular function, tissue metabolism and sufficient rest between loading, the body can adapt adequately.[1, 7, 25, 32]

It is important for healthy remodeling of a ligament or tendon that the fibers are laid down in proper alignment. Nonexcessive, well-directed loads on the structure with adequate rest encourage the healthy alignment of the fibers. The result is a structure that is stronger and also properly deformable, with adequate inter-fiber mobility. Good extensibility is also facilitated by remodeling with a normal ratio of collagen to ground substance. (It is important to have enough ground substance in the proportion.)[6, 23, 25] Production of ground substance is readily stimulated by movement after a ligament has been immobilized.[82]

There is now increasing evidence that connective tissues are equipped to repair themselves by manufacturing and remodeling large amounts of collagen and proteoglycans. These components are continuously, although slowly, remodeled in the tissue in its normal healthy condition. When an injury occurs, production of connective tissue (along with collagen and proteoglycans) can double or triple. Synthesis of collagen by the fibroblasts is given a high priority (for nutrient supply in the body) during the healing process. Fibroblasts are responsive to extra-cellular influences such as cytokines, growth factors and inflammatory mediators that allow fibroblasts to maintain and repair connective tissues. Fibroblasts are capable of proliferation to repopulate a region.[99]

Electricity, Magnetism, and Tendons/Ligaments

A number of researchers in the last three decades have found evidence demonstrating the presence and influence of electricity and magnetism in connective tissue function. This appears to have an effect on the health status of tendons and ligaments and their capacity for healing from injury.

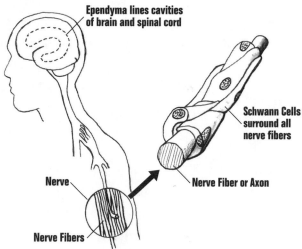

Orthopedic surgeon and researcher Robert Becker describes a bodily Direct Current system of internal communication, located in the perineural cells that ensheath the entire nervous system including the brain.[33, 34, 35] Becker traced the DC internal field map as it mirrors the design of the nervous system. This was confirmed by studies using the SQUID device for magnetic field detection.[33, 36, 37] It is an analog communication system that integrates body processes and controls the activity of the body's cells by producing DC electrical environments. The analog DC system is more primitive than the digital AC system of nerve impulse conduction, and can provide a relatively steady-state environment interacting with AC activity. Becker and others found this system to have an important role in growth and healing.[38, 39, 101]

FIGURE 6
Direct Current conduction system in perineural structures.

The Direct Current circuit flows appear to guide formation of collagen after tissue injury.[34] Dr. Becker describes a "current of injury" that is a DC flow from injured tissue that serves as a reporting mechanism. This conveys information of bodily damage to the brain and can evoke a response that is vital to reparative growth and other internal controls (see Figure 8). Magnetic energy was found to be increased at the location of injury.[33] The Swedish radiologist and researcher Nordenstrom also reports evidence demonstrating an electrical current circulatory system in the body switched on by infection and injury.[40] The cell biologist Lackie's research indicates that a wide variety of individual cells appear to have the ability to respond to DC fields.[41]

Williamson reports on tracing magnetic fields from the body that are produced by activity of potassium ions along cell membranes. He also asserts that ferromagnetic substances in the body can interact quite strongly with the geomagnetic field.[37] Becker reports on research showing the influence of the geomagnetic field on bodily growth patterns, stress responses, and biological cycles.[33, 34]

The physiologist and researcher Valerie Hunt describes a "growing emphasis from biomagnetic field studies on the electrical nature of life."[42] Motoyama and Reichmanis have both researched and demonstrated specialized electrical characteristics of the acupuncture meridian system.[40] Reichmanis found it to be linked to the perineural DC system and showed that acupoints generate DC potentials.[43] Hunt's research found acupuncture-like meridian energy flows in all connective tissue. She describes connective tissue as an anatomical electromagnetic circulatory system. The microtubular array of collagen in connective tissue is a structural component that facilitates this conduction.

Hunt's instrumentation detected differing electromagnetic currents in various body tissues. Denser tissue like bone and cartilage exhibited slower moving, lower frequencies that she associates more with direct current and magnetism. (This in comparison to "lighter" tissues like nerves and glands with higher frequencies and more alternating currents.) Tendons and ligaments as denser tissue exhibit the predominance of the magnetic part of the field.

Dr. Hunt characterizes the magnetic part of the spectrum as that which is instrumental in tissue healing.[42] She found that the energy at the location of an injury switches from predominantly electrical to become primarily magnetic in preparation for repair and healing. The increase of the low frequency magnetic field encourages repair cells to redifferentiate and grow. She notes the similarity of the repair role of this direct current flow to that which is described by Robert Becker. Hunt asserts that a primary breakdown in the body's healing response can occur in the electromagnetic system—in the strength and range of its impulses, as well as in its coherency. This appears to have a major influence on the condition and healing capacity of connective tissue including ligaments and tendons.

Contractile Capacity, Cellular Locomotion

Information that expands the conventional model until this point has been in the areas of neural involvement, bioelectromagnetism, and self-remodeling of the tissues. Another broadening of the perspective on the properties and functional capacity of connective tissue is provided by examining research on its contractile capacity and its cellular motility.

There is evidence for the widespread existence of the structural components and the active mechanism for contractile capacity in non-

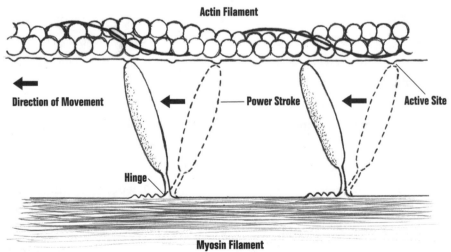

FIGURE 7
Acto-myosin motor

muscle cells. Cell biologists and biochemists have found a system of muscle-like proteins in nonmuscle cells, including fibroblasts. These proteins are actin, myosin, tropomyosin, and actinin. Actin is one of the body's most abundant proteins, constituting between 5 to 15 percent of the total protein content of cells.[2, 41, 44, 45] Actin can self-assemble into a helical polymer filament. Myosin is a hexamer and not a single protein.

The interaction between actin and myosin is basic to what is termed the *acto-myosin motor*, which is a primary contractile mechanism vital for muscle contraction. A primary component of this process is myosin filaments containing protruding heads, which are potential cross-bridges. The myosin heads fold/unfold as they attach and release by molecular bonding with various sites on the actin filament. This causes a pull that moves the actin. This contractile motor mechanism is found also in nonmuscle cells, including fibroblasts.[41, 45, 46, 47]

Cell locomotion occurs when the cell moves its position relative to its surroundings, and is the most sophisticated of cellular movements. Studies on tissue fibroblasts and large amoebae have provided much of the evidence for the mechanism of crawling movement of cells.[41, 44] The process includes a phase in which actin assembles into a cross-linked gel meshwork in the "front" or protrusive portion of the cell. This protruding region of the cell adheres to an anchorage beyond the present distal sites, so that the contractile machinery can pull the cell forward. Cell locomotion thus involves two main components: 1) the actomyosin motor system to generate contractile forces, and 2) an actin gel-assembly process for protrusion of the front of the cell. The cell surface must have the capacity for attachment, de-linking, and then reattachment to a new site.

Locomotion of fibroblasts is essential for wound-healing. The fibroblasts move into the area and then the contraction of numbers of fibroblasts pulls the edges of the wound together.[41, 44] Evidence for the mechanism of cellular contractile capacity and locomotor activity of nonmuscle cells, when applied to the fibroblasts of ligaments and tendons, indicates that these structures may not be as passive as was previously thought. Tendon and ligament tissue would possess the capacity to generate motion from within. This changes the perception of them as inert, passive structures that are only moved by external forces. The evidence would also indicate that the tissue has some capacity to reorganize itself into a different shape and to contract in ways that would facilitate the knitting together and condensing of tendons and ligaments that have been overstretched; these would have previously been considered to be permanently lax.

Possibilities for Tissue Regeneration in Tendons/Ligaments

To discover capabilities for tissue regeneration of injured tendons and ligaments, I have explored research findings for regeneration of various body structures; this provides a view into basic mechanisms of the process. There appear to be common features that are applicable to tendon and ligament healing. Extensive research in this area was done by Robert Becker in connection with his investigation of bioelectricity, but I will first discuss the regeneration and repair of muscle tissue by satellite cells.

The satellite cell in skeletal muscles was discovered by Mauro in 1950 and is the *stem cell* (unspecialized), which, when activated, provides a new cell population for muscle regeneration in vertebrates by transforming into myoblasts.[48] They are small mononuclear cells below the basement membrane, stored in the extra-cellular matrix of the muscle fiber.[49, 50] The Russian histology researcher Studitskii reports that "transformation of satellite cells into myoblasts is now an established fact."[50] This is particularly distinct following trauma, and may be instrumental in normal development and self-renovation of muscle fibers.[49, 51]

The two theories of satellite cell origin are: they are myonuclei that are pinched off from damaged muscle cells which then de-differentiate to form a population of myogenic cells, or they are an ongoing reserve

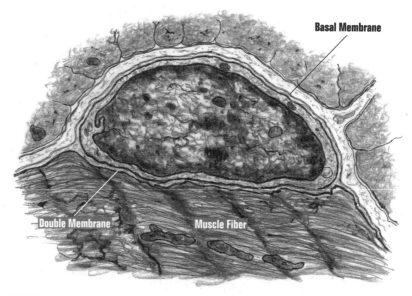

FIGURE 8
Satellite cell located in periphery of muscle fiber.

of precursor cells below the basement membrane.[52] They have the ability to synthesize DNA, divide, generate differentiating muscle cells, and give rise to new stem cells.[53] Under steady-state conditions stem cells are quiescent.[53] The result of satellite cell activation is development of daughter muscle fibers in maternal ones, and subsequent separation into new fibers. The molecular biologist and muscle researcher Richard Strohman reports that satellite cells can form new fibers or activate the thickening of existing fibers. This occurs not only after major damage, but in conditions of increased loading of the muscle where a normal repair function leads to strengthened fibers.[48, 49] He feels that normal growth and regeneration are different degrees of response along the same continuum.

Studitskii did extensive studies on skeletal muscle transplantation and grafting and the role of satellite cells. He defines plasticity as the capability for structural change depending on change of conditions. This is a different usage of the word from the description of "plastic range" of tissue deformability described earlier in this chapter. The plastic activity of muscle tissues is manifested by structural changes of growth and differentiation; it is facilitated by a particular reactive state of the tissue that Studitskii calls the *plastic state*.[50] The plastic state appears with any condition that deprives the muscle of its working capability, including weak traumatization. Plastic activity is a restorative phase that in muscles involves the appearance of satellite cells.[50]

My sense is that the concept of the plastic state and the conditions that favor it provide a very useful insight into successful strategies for connective tissue healing. There are some factors that *favor plastic activity* of muscle. These include hypervascularity (including ingrowth of blood vessels) and hyperinnervation of the tissue and surrounding areas. Activation of conditioned reflexes brought about by massage or exercise of the contralateral or adjacent muscles stimulates the plastic state.[50] Studitskii used various methods of interrupting the working activity of the muscle (including some irritants) to produce the state. Strohman finds that introducing a highly erratic stimulus activates stem cell growth.[49]

Passive stretch appears to be another facilitative influence on plasticity.[51] Both a high basal metabolic rate and adequate local tissue metabolism are helpful to plastic activity. Strohman reports his findings that local (hormonelike) growth factors in the tissue can activate satellite cell activity.[48] Studitskii emphasizes the importance of nerve influence (including trophic activity) for maintaining optimal metabolism of an organ or tissue and for facilitating the plastic state.[50]

Dr. Robert Becker's research findings on the perineural Direct Current system of control and communication in the body were described earlier. Here I present his findings on regenerative growth, mostly with electromagnetism in regeneration of limbs in vertebrates, and bone fracture healing in humans.[33, 34] He defines regeneration as the formation of complex body parts involving growth from simpler into more complex cells (redifferentiation). Physiological repair is defined as cell proliferation of the same type, which heals wounds by closing the gap. This is distinct from a wound being patched over with scar tissue.

Becker identifies two basic stages of regeneration. The first stage starts with wound clean-up, which culminates in the de-differentiation of nearby cells to form a blastema. A blastema is a mass of primitive embryonic cells appearing at the site of an injury. De-differentiation is the process in which a mature, specialized cell returns to its original, embryonic, unspecialized state, and apparently is stimulated by magnetic and DC flows after injury ("current of injury"). In the second phase also stimulated by DC flows, the embryonal cells pile up as the blastema elongates, and they then red-ifferentiate and take their proper place.[34]

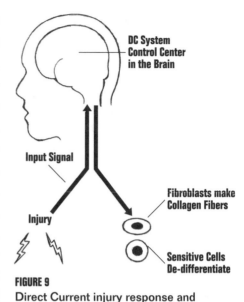

FIGURE 9
Direct Current injury response and growth control system.

Invertebrates can regenerate entire limbs. Becker theorizes that mammals cannot because they seem to lack two elements necessary for the first stage of regeneration (see above). One is that there is a shortage of cells sensitive enough to de-differentiate in order to form a blastema. The second element is that mammals lack a high enough ratio of nerve to limb tissue to produce adequate strength of the electrical stimulus needed for de-differentiation. However, he devised some successful strategies for facilitating the phases of regeneration in mammals by applied electromagnetism. This was particularly notable in facilitation of fracture healing in humans. Becker's research does show that collagen, so abundant in tendons and ligaments, is a piezo-electric generator, and also that collagen fibers can align in parallel in response to a weak DC flow. He feels that the potential repertoire of human cells is greater than is now realized and that there are possibilities for tissue regeneration that have not yet been actualized.[33, 34]

There are some important similarities in the findings concerning the essential features of tissue regeneration, when Becker's work is compared to that of the researchers on muscle regeneration involving satellite cells. Both approaches describe a process wherein there is cellular de-differentiation into unspecialized cells (or in some cases the appearance of unspecialized stem cells from other sources), which subsequently redifferentiate into specialized cells for tissue production and maintenance. The two lines of research have found that it is vital to have adequate nerve currents in the tissue. Both have also found that regeneration is favored by a healthy, strong metabolic function in the tissue, facilitated by adequate vascular and lymphatic flows. Although there hasn't been much focus in their work on tendon or ligament regeneration, Studitskii does mention findings that the localized fascias and tendons have a high degree of plasticity during muscle regeneration and that they repeatedly reorganize until a final structure is formed.[50]

A direct focus on connective tissue healing (and its involvement with cellular differentiation from simpler cells) is found in the work of the Danish cell biologist A. Viidik. His research indicates that connective tissue wound healing involves fibroblasts that are derived from undifferentiated perivascular mesenchymal cells, some of which come from the small blood vessels supplying the tendon or ligament.[26] Certain conditions that encourage the plastic state are available for tendons and ligaments, and would seem to favor their healing process. Viidik states that regeneration of the original tissues in connective tissue injury is not exceptional, and cautions not to assume that healing by scar tissue formation is the only possibility.[26]

Aside from the issue of cellular transformation, the fibroblasts themselves are active cells that can produce large amounts of collagen and ground substance. They are very active in wound healing and are capable of proliferation to repopulate a region.[99] Studitskii finds that fibroblasts play a major and essential role in the regeneration process.

An interesting perspective on the capabilities for tendon and ligament repair and regeneration is presented by the movement analyst, educator, and occupational therapist Bonnie Bainbridge Cohen. The educational/therapeutic approach she has developed, Body-Mind Centering, includes a segment of working with tendon and ligament problems; this reflects her view of these structures as being more responsive and functionally active than in the conventional model. Body-Mind Centering is empirically derived from 1) observation of sensing movement patterns and of clinical data, and 2) comparison of this with standard anatomical knowledge.[55] Regarding regeneration, Bainbridge Cohen believes that it is possible to reach a source of de-differentiated cells and activate them to effect de-differentiation.[56] She describes a structural matrix of the ligament that is comprised of small latticelike, electromagnetic hooklike connections. These "hook-ups" can realign into their innate pattern in response to therapeutic input, and effect significant tissue reorganization and healing.

She feels that overstretched, damaged tendons and ligaments can regain most or all of their proper tone, length, and thickness.[55] Their fibers can regain their proper spacing (proximity) and alignment. They can knit together, or loosen as needed. She states that conventional approaches have little idea of the actual possibilities for dramatic change of structure.[56]

Bonnie Bainbridge Cohen sees the role of ligaments as providing guidance, efficiency, and clarity to movement and alignment, and setting a pattern for muscular response.[55, 57] The ligaments provide an automatic movement control, and (as Basmajian also says) they fatigue more slowly than muscles, thus playing a vital role in weight-bearing and maintenance of posture.[21] Her view is that one can initiate movement from the tendons or ligaments, and that activating the ligaments adds to movement clarity and range. The activation will decrease muscular effort and tension. It is important to use the ligaments in movement. Body-Mind Centering uses a manual therapy approach that is extremely specific and detailed in its treatment of tendons and ligaments. She feels that there is some contractile capacity of their tissue and that they have a contractile function.[56, 57] Bainbridge Cohen's perspective is that the traditional view sees ligaments as too passive; they have a fuller, more active role and healing capacity.

Summary

Structure, properties, and function of tendons and ligaments are described in this chapter. I have illustrated the process of tendon/ligament injury and the anatomical and physiological changes in continuing dysfunction. The normal remodeling process of healthy connective tissue portrayed in this chapter is a foundation for the recovery process. One sees many of these elements at work in the situation of the dancer's tendon injury in Chapter 1 and in the cases of people to be reported later.

The standard medical view of ligaments is that they are passive rubber band-like structures. They are seen as "fixed-length stays" whose neural function consists of some proprioception and involvement in a simple reflex loop system that provides protection for the joint.

Research findings demonstrate that ligaments (and tendons) are more active structures having a significant role in weight-bearing and postural control, responsive to electrical and magnetic activity, and containing tissue components possessing some contractile capacity. These findings show a relatively extensive neural role for these structures with involvement in the gamma motor system and substantial provision of vital afferent input to the CNS. This is essential to coordination of movement and posture. Some functional aspects of ligaments seen in these research findings are favorable factors in potential for healing from injury.

The standard medical view of the injury healing capacity is that once it has been stretched beyond the limits of the plastic range, a ligament becomes permanently lax and cannot regain its normal tone and structure. A chronic injury consisting of a significant degree of fibrous rupture of a tendon or ligament is considered to have little or no possibility of recovery without surgical treatment. Surgery itself often does not have a favorable prognosis for promoting full recovery.

Increased healing capacity for tendons/ligaments is indicated in recent research. One can be encouraged by the chapter's evidence for the factors listed below.

Factors that enhance tendon/ligament repair described in this chapter appear to comprise a *basic bodily healing response* that may function in any area. These elements are reactions to injury, promoting the healing process. While many factors also may encourage recovery, the following list emerges from the research findings and theory in the preceding pages. A basic healing response for an injured structure is:

- appearance and/or proliferation of the types of cells in the injured tissue that are necessary for its repair. I have mentioned stem cell (less specialized) activation that leads to re-differentiation into specialized cells. Another possibility is proliferation of characteristic cells (e.g. fibroblasts) in the tissue.

- acceleration and intensification of normal tissue renovation and remodeling to restore a healthy structure (the proliferation of fibroblasts in response to injury mentioned above is one example of this mechanism in connective tissue).

- activity of hormonelike growth factors in the inflammation stage and repair process.

- electromagnetic activity involving an electrical current circulatory system (this may be a perineural Direct Current control system) responding with a "current of injury." This can guide tissue remodeling and encourage the reparative function of the cells.

- neural feedback circuits connect to the central nervous system and promote healthy autonomic and somatic neural control of metabolic and movement/postural activity for the injured area.

• the "plastic state" promotes tissue regeneration. Plasticity here is the capacity for structural change. This particular reactive state of the tissue appears in response to injury and in muscle involves activation of satellite (stem) cells. Plastic activity is facilitated by several factors including plentiful vascular and neural activity in the injury area, along with high basal metabolism and adequate local tissue metabolism.

In addition to the elements of a general healing response there are other specific factors that can promote tendon/ligament recovery. I have referred to contractile and locomotive capacity of some of their tissue components, along with connective tissue motility (generating of forces from within). The continuous metabolic turnover and remodeling process (self-renovation) of connective tissue are also health-enhancing influences, as is the effect of adequate neurotrophic supply of nutrients to the injury area.

Certain therapeutic strategies emerge from the referenced sources that would encourage the mechanisms that allow tendon and ligament healing. These can enhance all the processes I have described as elements of healing response. For the chronically injured structure the strategies are: a) to increase its oxygenation, b) to raise its metabolic rate (energy level of the tissue), c) ensure adequate vascular and lymphatic flow, d) reduce inflammation, e) normalize the electromagnetic climate of the body region, f) restore normal mechanics to the adjacent joints, g) establish normal, balanced patterns of afferent input from the joint and tendon/ligament, h) restore an adequate quantity of its ground substance (ratio of ground substance to fiber), i) re-establish the normal mobility and alignment of the individual fibers and their bundles. Chapter 5 depicts these and other anatomical/physiological changes occurring as the structure heals, as they relate to manual therapy.

Findings of the various scientific researchers in this chapter are a basis for its view of tendons/ligaments' favorable factors and capacities for recovery. This view points to greater possibility for their healing from chronic injury than in the conventional model. Expanded healing potential accords with research data and clinical theory of researcher-clinicians such as Becker, Bainbridge Cohen, Hunt, and Korr. The upcoming material on manual therapy and case study accounts will show how this chapter's capacities, favorable factors, and strategies can be utilized in a manual therapy approach to promote recovery.

CHAPTER 3

A Manual Therapy Model for Tendon and Ligament Injuries

In this chapter I will discuss: 1) the skills and aptitudes necessary for this approach; 2) the various manual therapy techniques that are used, including some unorthodox usages of these techniques specific to injury treatment that I have developed; 3) essential principles of the techniques; 4) comparison of my treatment model with the conventional medical methods, especially standard physiotherapy; 5) my personal background as it relates to the model. Initially, as a reference point to a new approach, I will outline the conventional medical treatment received by the majority of patients in this society.

Conventional Medical Treatment

Traumatic injury to a tendon or ligament is initially treated by rest, ice, compression, and elevation. Use of a splint will rest the tendon and thus promote healing. Nonsteroidal anti-inflammatory drugs such as aspirin, Ibuprofen, and others are used to reduce swelling. After the acute phase or in longer-term gradual onset injury, contrast baths with alternating warm water and cold water are employed to improve local circulation. Devices are used that limit the motion range of the structure (e.g. a heel lift to treat an Achilles tendon injury).[8]

As pain and swelling subside a stretching program for the injured structure is started, using both passive and active range of motion. Other physiotherapy procedures used are whirlpool baths, ultrasound, and electrical stimulation.[58, 60, 61, 100] Strength training for the neighboring muscles includes isometric and various forms of isotonic resistance exercise. Massage techniques can be used, including transverse friction (cross-fiber) for the tendon or ligament.[25, 62] Various forms of manual joint mobilization are sometimes performed by the physio-therapist.

Cortisone injections for the injured tendon or ligament are some-times utilized to reduce inflammation. There is some controversy around this procedure due to evidence that it causes atrophy of con-nective tissue and possible rupture of the tendon.[7, 14, 26, 63] Viidik states that use of anti-inflammatories, including corticosteroids, can be a cause of prolonged inflammation in connective tissue.[26]

Surgical techniques for musculoskeletal injuries can be categorized as either repair or removal. The orthopedic surgeon Garrick's view is that in general there is a higher success rate for removal operations, (e.g. removing bone spurs or fragments in a joint or thinning adhe-sions of an Achilles tendon sheath). Most surgeries for tendon or ligament injuries are repairs.[7, 8, 15] In describing reconstruction surg-eries for damaged anterior cruciate ligaments of the knee, Seedhom mentions: 1) primary repairs, 2) reconstruction with different tissues, 3) reconstruction with various synthetic devices.[11]

Frankel describes various forms of primary repair surgeries in which the tendon or ligament fibers are woven together. The end-weave method, which is strongest, has the disadvantage of being bulkier and possibly inhibiting gliding on adjacent structures.[7] In reconstruc-tion using natural tissue, those used are: autogenous tissue (e.g. tissue from the patient's iliotibial band or patellar tendon for ACL repair), allografts using tissue grafted from a cadaver, or xenografts from bovine tissue. Repairs with synthetic materials use polyethylene, polypropy-lene, and carbon fiber. The synthetic repair can be a complete replace-ment, a supplement to a natural tissue graft, or a scaffolding that encourages ingrowth of the patient's collagen tissue.[11] While many patients have been returned to their accustomed activities by these repairs and there is often at least a short-term relief of discomfort, Garrick states that after surgery a tendon or ligament never recovers completely and that some don't recover at all.[15] Problems with the mobility and neuromuscular integration of the neighboring joint can be short-term or long-term consequences of the surgery.[1, 64] Recovery procedures from surgery consist of a period of immobilization followed by the treatment procedures previously described.

Skills and Aptitudes

Illustrating my therapeutic approach starts here with important abilities that are involved. This section describes these skills and aptitudes, often referring to the statements of some prominent osteopaths and allied practitioners. They are abilities that in my experience make it possible to effectively practice the techniques that are presented in the next section.

It is very beneficial to be capable of detecting small bodily changes and picking up strains at "micrometric levels" of measurement.[65, 66] This involves the perception of bodily movements from the smallest and most simple, to the most complex.[67] One detects a difference between old and new strains.[66] There is the capacity to detect and become attuned to the rhythms of the patient's body (e.g. breathing, Cranial Rhythmic Impulse), some of which are quite subtle.[68, 69]

A thorough knowledge of anatomy and kinesiology is indispensable to me. The practitioner needs a familiarity with the normal motions of the body,[67] a clear image of the normal joint articulations and their mechanics, and a knowledge of the position and purpose of each structure. This familiarity, combined with an understanding of body structure and function, enables the effective and useful comparison of the normal body with the abnormal,[70] and the interpretation of material into sound physiological reasoning.[66]

It is important to be able to establish contact with the body while disturbing its function as little as possible.[71] Developing the capacity of using a very light, neutral touch is favorable for fine perception, allowing both information and therapeutic change to come through to my hands rather than pushing to discern something in the tissues or to force changes.[69] One allows the body to give its opinion,[66] as restrictions in the body may literally attract the hand to them—and take the practitioner to the center of dysfunctioning patterns.[72] Sutherland, who originated osteopathic cranial therapy, advises the therapist to develop familiarity with using the least force possible to accomplish the objective.[73] Skill enables accuracy, as Barral states; only very slight forces are needed for effecting structural change when one is precise.[72]

There is a skill in being able to synchronize one's attention. While I am working, the aim of internal physical focus is a state of attentive, balanced relaxation throughout my body, including all the senses. The osteopath Jealous calls this "defacilitation" of the practitioner's CNS, which involves relaxed breathing and muscular relaxation.[68] Centering within the practitioner's own body enables attunement to the patient's rhythm. Magoun calls this meditation-like state "a rapport in the tissues between practitioner and patient."[71]

Bainbridge Cohen speaks of the capacity to direct or focus one's sense organs. Sensing and perceiving are not just passively receiving input, but when done with attention and discriminatory awareness, become a "dynamic activeness of perceiving."[57] Rollin Becker advises developing a "listening finger-touch," which is more than a passive laying-on of hands—becoming an alert, observational type of awareness.[66] This capacity of "listening," an active receptivity, is a vital element of my work that is integrated into every aspect of diagnosis and treatment.

The practitioner develops the sensitivity of the sensory receptors (mentioned in Chapter 2) of his hand. The potential sensitivity of the human hand to pressure, motion, and heat is extremely high, and far greater than usually realized.[74, 82] Mechanoreceptors, proprioceptors and temperature sensors respond to these stimuli as well as to vibration.[68] Barral asserts that there is considerable evidence for palpation of infrared radiation (heat), and concurs with Hunt that receptors in the hand are sensitive to a wide variety of electromagnetic wavelengths.[42, 74] It is very useful for the therapist to be able to perceive and interact with various aspects of the electromagnetic field of the patient. The hand's receptors are located in skin, deep fascia, in and around joints (ligaments, tendons), and in muscle spindles.

The references quoted in this section from these leading teachers demonstrate much of the "lineage" of my model. This proceeds from the pioneering Sutherland and Lippincott, who incorporated A.T. Still's beginnings of osteopathy, up to the present-day teachers who are quoted. These include Smith, with a direction from Chinese medicine, and Bainbridge Cohen, whose work stems from earlier movement educators such as Bobath and Todd.

To conclude with the aptitudes: it is important that the clinician can sense and encourage motion and mobility within the tissues as initiated by these living structures[66]—realizing that manipulation is no substitute for the body's own power.[67] I have endeavored to follow in the style of treatment based on the principle of osteopathy being the art of provoking self-correction on the part of the organism.

Techniques I Use for Tendon/Ligament Treatment

The principal methods in my model are the osteopathic techniques of Strain/Counterstrain, Cranial therapy, and Visceral Manipulation, combined with techniques from Body-Mind Centering. Their active use is seen in the injury cases to be reported. There is also a significant role for acupressure, Zero Balancing, and osteopathic Fascial/Myofascial Release techniques. This section will describe the basic mechanism and features of each technique and discuss how I use it to address various aspects of tendon/ligament injury. Chapter 5 also relates these therapies to the specific processes and tissue changes that occur in injury healing.

Strain/Counterstrain, one of the major osteopathic manual therapy techniques, was originated by Dr. Lawrence Jones starting in the early 1960s.[28, 64, 75] I have made extensive use of it since 1977. It is a gentle atraumatic technique that ameliorates joint dysfunction through the use of positional release. I move the patient's body slowly in nonpainful

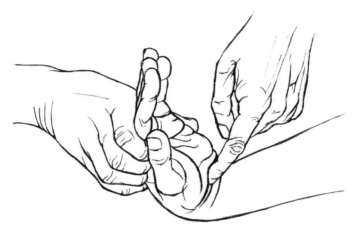

FIGURE 10
One of the Counterstrain techniques for the carpal joints involves positioning the wrist primarily in flexion, while monitoring the decrease of localized tension and soreness in the indicator ("tender") point under the therapist's finger. The weight of the subject's hand and arm is thoroughly supported to relax in the position of release.

directions, guided by local decrease in tissue tension and palpatory tenderness (in an indicator or "tender" point) under my monitoring hand, to find the optimal position of release. The patient is supported in this position of comfort for ninety seconds. It is usually an exaggeration of an abnormal alignment pattern, and involves the purposeful shortening of one or more tense muscles around the problematic joint.

As I locate and maintain the exact release position, the tense hypersensitive tissue near the joint feels like it softens and loosens. There is a sense of activation and an even current (of electricity and acupuncture energy) moving under my monitoring hand. Often, I palpate an activation of localized vascular pulsation that after some seconds becomes more quiet and even.

The positioning effects the reduction and arrest of inappropriate (excessive) proprioceptor activity by markedly shortening muscles that contain habitually overactive muscle spindle (stretch) receptors. This quiets afferent discharge from the spindle (as well as other mechanoreceptors in tendon/ligament or fascia) and normalizes the alpha-gamma loop firing pattern; that enables the balancing of muscular and other soft tissue forces around the joint which is being treated.[16] The gamma loop is discussed in Chapter 2 (see Figure 4). The positioning influences the CNS to gradually turn down the "alarm signal" level of gamma efferent discharge to the affected muscle, allowing the muscle to regain its normal resting length. This repatterning of local and regional neural and soft tissue activity enables the joint to regain healthy alignment and motion. I have found the technique to be very advantageous in treating a wide variety of spinal and other joint-related dysfunctions.

The use of Counterstrain technique specifically benefits an injured tendon or ligament by reducing excessive muscular pulls on it—as well as reducing pulls from fascial tensions, structural misalignment, and pressure on Golgi tendon receptors. My experience is that because it is so gentle, the technique is very helpful for treating fragile, injured, or hyper-reactive areas. Reduced tissue stress in the area leads to reduction of inflammatory fluid and improvement of fluid dynamics and metabolic activity.

The positionings also promote recovery by improving mobility and usage patterns of the joint (near that ligament) through normalizing patterns of afferent input and balancing ligamentous pulls on all sides of the joint. The employment of Counterstrain corrections of (spinal) segmental dysfunction reduces or eliminates the output of neural misinformation; this neural output involves reflexes to the CNS and also involves irritated mechanoreceptors and nociceptors in a tendon or ligament which is in that segmental circuit. In treatment of a tendon/ligament injury I have used Counterstrain and related positionings that shorten the injured structure to more effectively perform specific tissue work with it while it is in the shortened position (see the following description of Body-Mind Centering techniques). This seems to reduce excessive localized proprioceptor activity in the tendon, which effects change in itself and enables greater efficacy of other techniques that I am using while the tendon is in that position.

The therapeutic model of *cranial osteopathy* is based on the existence of an active, mobile cranio-sacral system consisting of the cranial bones and membranes, the spine and its membranes, and the cerebrospinal fluid. Originated by Sutherland in the early years of this century, the model includes the twenty-two bones of the cranium having joints with a slight mobility—and a reciprocal tension membrane system consisting of the spinal membranes connecting with the intra-cranial membranes. The therapy is described in works by Sutherland,[73] Magoun,[71] Frymann,[76] and Gehin.[77] There is a characteristic dual-phased motion pattern of the cranio-sacral system (cranial rhythmic impulse, or CRI) that is normally six to twelve cycles/minute. My work with the rhythmic fluctuations of this system (and its wavelike movement that is reflected through the whole body) is both diagnostic and therapeutic.

Restrictions and imbalances of the cranial structure are treated with gentle manual techniques, often consisting of the indirect approach. Indirect technique consists of encouraging the structural compo-nents in a direction exaggerating the existing imbalance by following the mechanical pulls and forces of that body region to what feels to me like a point of rest; this allows rebalancing and improved condition of the localized structure. Indirect technique is also utilized in Counterstrain and to some extent in all other methods that I employ. Also similar to Counterstrain is the basic premise of inherent self-corrective forces in the body; the body is a self-correcting organism.

My therapeutic usage of cranial osteopathy for tendon and liga-ment injuries includes the harmonizing of a peripheral structure (such as a ligament) with the CNS through connections to the spine and cra-nium. For an injured hand ligament this strategy involves my freeing the motion of the CRI to that ligament through the upper limb—connecting from the dural membrane of the lower cervical spine (from which the ligament derives innervation).

Another example of benefit for an injury would be the freeing of a cranial structure such as the occipito-mastoid suture, having a ben-eficial effect on membranous tension in the upper spine, which connects to fascial tensions going through to the ligament in the hand. The usage of fascial unwinding (described later here) is included in cranial therapy. In a more general sense, alleviating excessive tensions

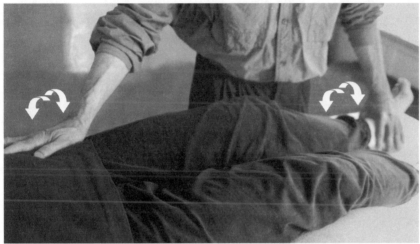

FIGURE 11

A technique for working with the dual-phased movement of the cranial rhythmic impulse (CRI) through the hip to the ankle and foot. Using gentle pressures the therapist balances and synchronizes the CRI movements (arrows) of external and internal rotation of the hip, connecting to the lower spine—with the CRI motion in the ankle and foot. This method is used to synchronize motion through an injured Achilles tendon in a case study in Chapter 4.

in the cranium and spine relieves pressures on important neural structures, which may effect changes such as reduction of excessive sympathetic nervous system activity. This reduction can lead to improved circulation to the body periphery where an injured tendon is located.[64]

Bonnie Bainbridge Cohen's theoretical and clinical model of the role and healing capacity of tendons and ligaments has been described in the second chapter. Her system of movement analysis and training, anatomy/kinesiology education, and manual therapy is called Body-Mind Centering, and has been developed since the early 1970s. The foundation of Body-Mind Centering (BMC) is the exploration and repatterning of the major body systems (skeletal, muscular, organ, endocrine, nervous, and fluid) as they initiate and support movement.[57]

Her experience as an occupational therapist leads to this method's focus on neurodevelopmental movement patterns. Optimal structural alignment is promoted in relation to the movement repatterning. In practicing this technique the therapist aims to utilize a level of sensing and activation of structures (including tendons and ligaments) down to their

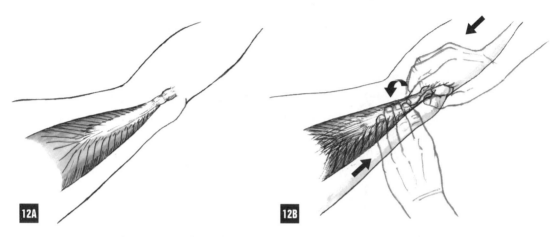

FIGURES 12A, 12B, AND 12C
Feeding in ends of a tendon alternated with drawing them apart. Therapy for a biceps femoris tendon injury was described in Chapter 1, and this technique encourages proper alignment of its fibers. Figure 12A shows the tendon before treatment, with its adhesions and misalignment near the knee. Figures 12B and 12C illustrate the feeding in phase of condensing the fibers longitudinally, which allows re-organization (see below). At the same time, the right hand is also used here with rotation to specifically aid re-alignment of a portion of the tendon which was particularly twisted (using indirect technique).

more minute components (e.g. fibers). This fine perception and control is utilized clinically in the BMC manual therapy approach to tendon and ligament injuries that is the most structurally specific and complete of any that I have encountered.[55, 56, 57, 78] I have made extensive use of it since 1974.

I use the BMC manual method of contacting both ends of a ligament (a similar method contacting the bony insertion and musculotendinous junction for a tendon), and alternately feeding these ends in towards each other and drawing them apart. For a shortened, thickened ligament my emphasis would be more in the drawing apart phase, and more on feeding in for a lax, weak ligament.

When a tendon is too short, separating the fibers perpendicular to their length will allow it to elongate. When it is weak and lax, unifying the fibers will allow it to condense. I alternate separating and con-

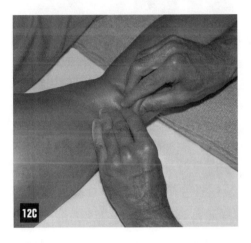

densing the fibers width-wise (perpendicularly) as well as longitudinally. This involves activation of what Bainbridge Cohen believes to be the perpendicular component of the microstructure of the tendon.

Bainbridge Cohen feels that tendon or ligament fibers naturally organize their structural interrelation with neighboring fibers by a "hooking" mechanism that creates a structural integrity. By manually condensing the ligament (longitudinally) one disorganizes the misaligned fibers and encourages this self-generated hooking activity. The result is that the fibers are allowed to assume their natural organization. I find this similar to, and compatible with, the Counterstrain approach of placing the ligament in a shortened position. For a lax and weakened ligament I position the joint so the ligament is shortened, and concurrently use direct manual contact with it to specifically encourage its fibers in knitting together and increasing its tone.

Additional clinical strategies of BMC that can be used for tendon/ligament injuries include a subtle manual contact through tissue layers to the capillaries in the area, in order to encourage healthy vascular flow in the tendon and its surroundings. This is done through gentle pumping action, which has the added effect of stimulating movement of the interstitial fluids in the localized zone.

Repair is also enhanced by lessening strain patterns in bones adja-

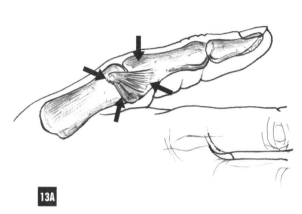

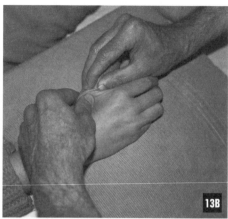

FIGURES 13A, 13B, AND 13C
BMC techniques for increasing tone and substance, and decreasing laxity of the ulnar collateral ligament of the MP joint (seen in a later case study). The therapist is condensing the ligament from both ends as well as in a perpendicular direction. The schematic drawings (13C) show the ligament before treatment and then as it is being condensed.

cent to the injury area using BMC induction-type techniques; trauma or repetitive stresses can cause the various layers of bone to retain compaction and torquing that contribute to the unbalanced pulls on nearby structures. The clinician aims to activate direct movement initiation and create feedback and proprioception in the ligament. This activation of movement initiation in the injured structure is encouraged by the client's gentle movement of the adjacent joint, while I am focusing the movement in the ligament and offering a slight resistance. Resistance up to a certain level (and no more) will increase proprioception. The specificity and structural insight of Bainbridge Cohen's approach is of great value for my treatment of some fragile and stubborn connective tissue problems.

The osteopathic *Visceral Manipulation* techniques described and taught by Jean-Pierre Barral also aim at the normalization of reciprocal tensions throughout the body (as do all the techniques in the model). This includes some very effective assessment methods of "listening" for identifying the center(s) of these tensions. The treatments are focused on optimizing the structural condition and move-

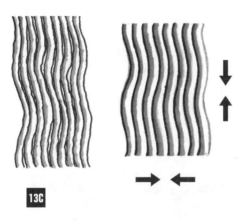

ment patterns of the organs of the pelvis, abdomen, and thorax.[67, 68, 79, 80, 81] Effective usage of Visceral Manipulation incorporates Barral's emphasis on anatomical precision. The techniques are direct and indirect low-force methods for freeing restrictions of the organs and their adjacent and surrounding connective tissues. These organs are structurally and functionally interrelated with the rest of the body through the fascial system and fluid and nerve pathways. It has often been my experience that a visceral restriction contributes significantly to a client's musculo-skeletal problem (e.g. lumbo-sacral dysfunction) and that improvement of the visceral motion will result in definite benefit for the spinal problem.

Some examples of the method's use for tendon and ligament injuries are as follows: in addressing injuries in the upper limb I have often found it very helpful to use Barral's techniques for freeing the upper lobe of the lung, its pleura, and the strong connective tissue attachments of the pleura to the first rib, T1, and lower cervical spine[79, 81] (see Figures 14A and 14B). Injuries in the lower limb (e.g. Achilles tendon) seem to derive benefit if the clinician can free a lower abdominal/pelvic restriction such as limited mobility of the cecum or sigmoid colon. The general and local "listening" diagnostic methods in which the therapist allows his hand to be attracted and led to the important restriction are quite useful to me in clearly identifying regional structural dysfunctions in the tendon or ligament area.

Visceral Manipulation uses the technique of induction, in which the operator gently encourages the structural component(s) in the direction of ease, least resistance, and greater motion, until a point of equilibrium is reached—and is then maintained until a release occurs in that structure (see Figure 14B). I have used induction (an indirect technique) to advantage in tendon treatment by following the pulls in the tendon fibers, and find this to aid in the correction of their alignment pattern. The technique responds to, and works to balance, the major force vectors in the tissues. It works to promote their balance and lessen their disrupting influence.

The acupuncture system of Chinese medicine includes a grid of

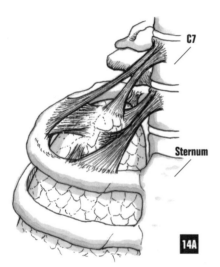
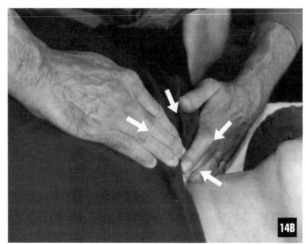

FIGURES 14A AND 14B
Technique for freeing restrictions of the upper lobe of the right lung, its pleura, and the connective tissue suspension of the top of the pleura. The clavicle is removed in Figure 14A to show the pleura's suspensory apparatus, which is being gathered by the therapist's left hand in Figure 14B. This induction technique is assisted here by the right hand's influence of slackening the tissue superiorly from below. The relaxed tissue may then exhibit pulls in various directions, which can be followed by the practitioner's hands.

energy pathways throughout the body called meridians. The acupuncture points on these meridians have been found to be zones of lowered electrical resistance.[40, 43, 83] Acupressure therapy was the initial study in my career, and I now utilize it most often as a background to the structural work that I do. However, there are times that I use it as a primary focus, and some of these are for tendon/ligament injuries. I find the meridian map very useful for discerning and treating restrictions and blockages that are connected to the injured structures. Applying pressure on acupuncture points in the localized area (sometimes connected with pressure on distant points) facilitates the normalization and smooth flow of electrical and magnetic activity and current in the tendon.

Acupressure is also involved in the manual therapy system called *Zero Balancing*, originated by the osteopath Fritz Smith in the 1970s.[69, 82] He is also an acupuncturist, and has blended the two approaches to create a type of structural acupressure. The system is designed to free and enhance the movement of the *ch'i* energy through the body structure. This acupuncture energy flow has an electrical component, and I have found Zero Balancing useful in working with the electrical activity in tendons and ligaments. In Dr. Smith's model, the densest energy flow comes through the bones and the body's energy is most readily blocked at the joints.

The techniques apply sustained pressures ("fulcrums") and tractions (applied "vectors") designed to rebalance joints by interrupting their neurological feedback to the CNS and removing their blockages. Zero Balancing is focused on the clear identification of acupuncture energy movement, and enhancement of its flow through the joints (where tendons and ligaments are located). In my experience it is an effective systematic approach for combining beneficial structural change with normalization of acupuncture/electrical current. I have found that Smith's methods are useful as alternatives to, and combinations with, the Counterstrain joint positionings and can be very helpful for freeing joint restrictions in the locality of tendon/ligament injuries.

Many of the fascial planes of the body intersect at joints and I have found it essential to free the fascias in order to relieve excessive pulls and pressures on injured structures. All the techniques mentioned so far accomplish this to some extent, but I will now describe a specific method for addressing the fascias. I use osteopathic *Fascial Release* techniques, which also effect more optimal fluid and nerve function in the tendon or ligament by relieving strain on the fascial wrapping of vessels and nerves.[84, 85] The three major varieties of fascia (superficial, deep and subserous) form an interconnected reciprocal tension meshwork, which is the packing and wrapping of structures throughout the body.[5, 30, 85] The deep fascia can develop the most stubborn restrictions,

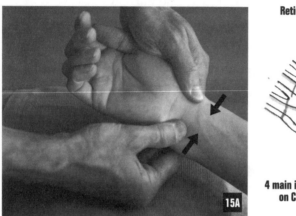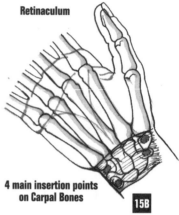

FIGURES 15A, 15B, 16A, AND 16B
Fascial Release (indirect technique) can be used in combination with direct technique of stretching for the interosseus membrane, similarly for the flexor retinaculum of the wrist, which forms a boundary of the carpal tunnel. Figure 15A of the retinaculum shows it being condensed as one component of a Fascial Release technique. Figure 16A of the membrane portrays a direct stretch.

as it is the densest layer. This deep layer forms the sheaths for tendons and ligaments.

Fascial Release Technique[84] is based on the principle of evaluating motion (of a joint or soft tissue) in all three planes and carrying it in the combined direction(s) of most freedom to a position of rest. The rest position is maintained until inherent movement restarts (or is subtly encouraged in the direction of ease), and the clinician follows in this direction with gentle manual pressure until there is balanced, free motion. This process is sometimes called fascial unwinding. In the course of freeing the restrictions of these tissues I find that there is sometimes also a release of memories and emotions associated with the physical pattern. This associated "tissue memory" is a common occurrence in the aftermath of high-impact injuries and its release can be helpful to the recovery process. I often combine Fascial Release (indirect) technique with direct techniques of stretching the fascial structures. The direct technique is very useful for zones of stubborn fascial binding and adhesion. It has been of vital importance for injury

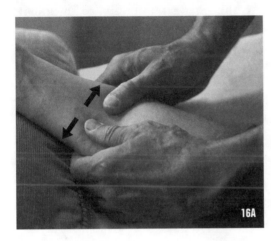

16A

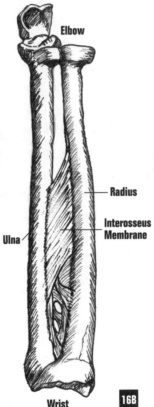

Elbow

Radius

Interosseus
Membrane

Ulna

Wrist   16B

treatment to free the fascias, including the periosteum, in the close vicinity of the tendon/ligament.

These techniques that I employ for treating the fascias are also very useful for *freeing restrictions in* the *muscles.* There is much structural interconnection: with perimysium wrapping bundles of muscle fibers, endomysium wrapping individual fibers, reticula entering the fiber, and septas separating groups of muscles. This configuration allows Fascial Release technique to be used efficaciously for muscle treatment, and it may appropriately be termed myofascial release.

The Golgi tendon organs near the musculotendinous junctions respond to changes in force (tension).[16, 86] Stimulation of these receptors effects an inhibiting neural influence on muscle contraction and causes the muscle to relax. I use the technique from Applied Kinesiology[86] in which the therapist applies direct pressure to the Golgi tendon organ to relax the attached muscle and return it to a more optimal resting length.

A crucial element of the recovery process is the relaxation of excessive muscle tensions that place abnormal strain on injured ligaments and tendons. This is accomplished by my use of the Fascial Release techniques, Golgi tendon organ pressures, and also by Counterstrain positionings. As described earlier in this chapter, the positioning shortens the muscle, relieving aberrant neuromuscular strain patterns, which allows it to then assume a more relaxed resting length.

Methods that I use for promoting normal, harmonious electromagnetic activity include manual pressure on certain acupressure points in the injury area and in areas adjacent to it. The smooth flow of electricity and magnetism is also facilitated by the cranial therapy approach of working with the CRI movement through the area of the tendon or ligament—sometimes connecting this all the way through to the spine and cranium.

I have developed a specific method of normalizing *electromagnetic activity* that consists of my feeling to discern if there is any sense of a blocked and overactive ("dammed-up") or a deficient electrical quality in the tendon. This can feel like the discontinuity and unevenness of "static" or uneven magnetic pulls. I then move the tendon tissue a small distance, to the placement that encourages smooth electrical current that flows through it freely in an increasingly steady, unpressured pattern. This placement also effects a sense of balanced, even magnetic pulls in the tendon. The positioning (which can be readjusted in the process of change) often involves condensing of the tendon or ligament fibers.

Electrical activity can also be balanced through applying manual contact on either side (proximally and distally) of a ligament or tendon. The therapist then applies a slight traction, compression, or rotational force between the two hands until the intervening flow of electrical current through the ligament is smooth, even, and balanced from one hand to the other. Another option is to apply mild direct, localized pressure to the ligament tissue until electrical (and/or magnetic) activity is balanced.

Some general findings are that weak, deficient activity often can be strengthened and increased by a light, shaking movement applied to the area, or stretching of the skin over the ligament. Tonification is also achieved by contact on either side (proximal and distal) that is used to apply a compression force by approximating my two hands (or fingers). Calming of "jangled," overactive electricity or magnetism in the ligament is promoted by applying mild traction through the area

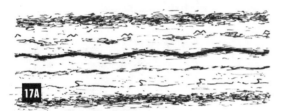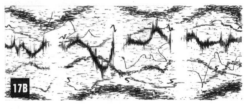

FIGURES 17A AND 17B
Electrical activity in a ligament. Figure 17A is of balanced, even current and 17B of disrupted, noncoherent current. These illustrations are not numerical measurements. They represent a palpatory sense of this activity felt with my hands through manual contact with the ligament.

or applying gentle localized pressure to the tissue. These general guidelines may vary in different situations. When there is much compaction and tension in the tissue, one may need to begin by shortening it with contact from both ends (condensing) before traction can be applied.

The sensation of electrical activity is often a tingling, humming, or buzzing feeling of the current. The sensations I discern of magnetic activity in the tissue are somewhat similar, with more of a "pulling" quality. Magnetism is usually sensed as a slower movement/activity than the electricity in the area.

The normal electrical pattern of a tendon/ligament is experienced as predominately linear. This may correspond to their parallel fiber arrangement and adaptation to tensile forces. In comparison, the pattern of current through a visceral structure such as the stomach is more diffuse, with more of a rotational component.

In regard to the capacity of the human hand to detect a variety of electromagnetic frequencies, I have already mentioned the assertion of this aptitude by the researcher-clinicians Barral, Hunt, and Smith.[42, 74, 82] Studies by researchers such as Motoyama, Reichmanis, and Becker demonstrate that the current of the acupuncture system through the points of the meridians has an electromagnetic component (see Chapter 2). Acupuncturists for many centuries have been perceiving the fluctuation of this current in their diagnosis and treatment. The acupuncturist-physician Helms states that acupuncture treatment activates electromagnetism in the body including localized ionic migration in the interstitial fluid as well as fascial

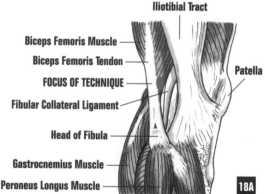

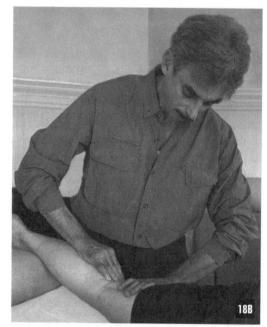

Iliotibial Tract

Biceps Femoris Muscle

Biceps Femoris Tendon

FOCUS OF TECHNIQUE

Fibular Collateral Ligament

Patella

Head of Fibula

Gastrocnemius Muscle

Peroneus Longus Muscle

18A

18B

FIGURES 18A AND 18B
Work with weakened, damaged zone of left hamstring tendon. Left hand is gathering surrounding structures in direction of zone at tips of 2nd and 3rd fingers of right hand. Right hand anchors and supports distal portion of tendon, and is also in position for specific fiber work with the localized zone. Figure 18A shows a normal hamstring tendon (right leg), indicating the zone being addressed in Figure 18B.

and perineural semiconduction throughout the body.[98] My experience is that as I detect the electrical current in a body area becoming more even and steady, the tissue exhibits relaxation of excessive tension and improved vascular flow.

This section on methods has included description of how these techniques can at times be combined for benefiting tendons and ligaments. My feeling is that while this can be quite valuable, it is not a substitute for learning one or more of the techniques thoroughly.

Essential Principles of the Techniques

There are some common essential principles of the techniques in the preceding section. These principles are:

- Normalizing force patterns and reciprocal tension pulls in the body—combined with precise attention to localized centers of dysfunction and stress.

- Harmonizing the peripheral structures (i.e. tendon/ligament) with the center of the body and CNS (through the vertebral column and cranium).

- Re-establishing movement that is balanced and unobstructed is basic to (structural) health.

- There are intrinsic movement and force patterns in the body (i.e. CRI and optimal fluid circulation). Facilitating these patterns to operate freely is beneficial.

- Encouraging self-correction in the body. This is founded on a belief in the intelligence of the body, down to its minute components. When given the opportunity, it is a self-correcting organism.

- Usage of small, well-targeted changes (e.g. at the foci of physiological patterns) can have a major impact when the clinician comprehends the overall structure and dynamic.

- Combination of direct and indirect approach, with extensive usage of indirect techniques, in which the therapist follows the body's structural and movement inclination.

Comparison of My Therapeutic Model for Tendon/ Ligament Injuries with Conventional Medical Treatment

This comparison for my approach is to the conservative care in the conventional model (standard physiotherapy and medication). I do incorporate some aspects of the standard approach that are useful. The prevalent physiotherapy modalities that can be beneficial are heat/cold applications, stretching/strengthening exercise, electro-stimulation devices ("electro-stim"), ultrasound, and sometimes use of braces and splints. All of these except electro-stim and ultrasound are used for home-care procedures by the subjects in the case studies. Occupational therapy can be beneficial in providing tools, mechanical aids, and retraining body usage patterns to minimize injury aggravation. Prescription and nonprescription anti-inflammatory drugs can accomplish temporary changes (in serious cases) that fit into a treatment program.

The standard medical treatment for tendons and ligaments seems to be quite useful in some less serious injuries, and has aspects that are useful in all levels of injury. However, in general it does not seem to be designed for actually reversing serious, chronic injuries with major tissue damage. As described in an earlier section of this chapter, the conceptual model it employs does not include much possibility of full recovery with conservative care, of that level of tendon/ligament injury.

While some physiotherapists have trained beyond the standard approach, the comparison to my model that I will be making here is to this most prevalent (standard) approach, which is received by most patients. The various forms of heat/cold therapy, ultrasound, and electro-stimulation utilized in physiotherapy are all helpful for increasing circulation and oxygenation, reducing inflammation, and raising the metabolic rate of the tissue. These effects are not likely to be long-lasting in the absence of the following additional processes and changes: reduction of reciprocal tension pulls on the ligament involving body alignment patterns, normalization of neural activity, reduction of excessive cross-linkage, improvement of joint condition, and proper alignment of the fibers. These additional changes are promoted in my treatment.

Ultrasound is employed to lessen muscle tensions and has some effect of reducing adhesions. Again, however, these changes are not as complete or long-lasting in the absence of reduction of excessive, inappropriate proprioceptor activity (this is essential in the muscle spindles—see Counterstrain description) for change in the muscle condition, and in the absence of thorough reduction of reciprocal tension (e.g. fascial) pulls on localized tissue adhesions. These additional, crucial changes are accomplished with skilled manual therapy, which can also be considerably more precise and thorough in locating and treating adhesions (e.g. BMC, Fascial Release).

T.E.N.S. and other electro-stimulation devices can be used to reduce muscle spasm and alleviate pain, which reduces neural stress. The benefits of this modality are limited in their duration and their overall extent in similar ways to ultrasound and heat/cold therapy. The additional processes and changes (promoted by skilled manual therapy), which are needed for the other modalities, are also necessary for electro-stim to have more extensive and longer-lasting effects. In summary, the modalities of heat/cold therapy, ultrasound, and electro-stim are all useful in various ways, but on their own do not seem capable of accomplishing the major changes needed to reverse chronic and serious tendon/ligament injury. They can be employed as a part of an effective treatment for serious injury.

The stretching (active and passive) employed in physiotherapy can be useful to lessen muscular and fascial tensions, promote adequate extensibility of the tendon, and reduce adhesion. However, it is a very delicate and often problematic procedure to stretch a weakened tendon or ligament that has had much fibrous rupture. Resistance exercises for increasing strength are important for improving stability, and need to be used with the appropriate timing and level of exertion. Strengthening procedures will allow a tendon to gain better tone only when it does not have too much tissue damage. Their improper use can easily increase existing neurological and fibrous imbalances in injured structures.

Common manual therapy procedures of standard physical therapy are massage, joint mobilization, and cross-fiber massage. These methods can promote some of the important beneficial changes for tendon/ligament recovery when the operator is very skilled. However, in general, the massage approach seems to be mostly focused on treating standard patterns of muscle groups and not on locating and addressing necessary changes in specific concentrations of fascial restriction. Joint mobilization improves the mobility of the joint, but it can be problematic to use this degree of force in the area of an inflamed ligament with considerable tissue damage, which could cause exacerbation (indirect techniques, e.g. Counterstrain, would usually be more beneficial in this situation). The cross-fiber technique breaks down adhesion (depending on its orientation) but is often vigorous enough to cause irritation; it is often not very precise about bringing the fibers into proper alignment.

These common manual physiotherapy procedures do not specifically effect strengthening and increasing the substance of a weak, lax structure (see BMC technique description). There is not as much attention paid to alignment patterns in the tissues in relation to the nervous system. In comparison with the osteopathic techniques that I use, the standard approach does not incorporate as much of a whole-body methodology that is needed to harmonize the periphery with the spine, CNS and other parts of the body core (e.g. cranial therapy), and to reduce more distant reciprocal tension pulls on the tendon/ligament (cranial therapy, Visceral Manipulation). Neurological imbalances such as inappropriate gamma-loop functioning are more directly addressed with Counterstrain technique.

In speaking about manual physiotherapy I am generalizing and describing the most prevalent situation. Some physical therapists have altered and expanded this approach, and employ a variety of other techniques, including osteopathic methods. This comparison of my manual therapy treatment of tendons/ligaments is to the widely used physiotherapy in conventional medical treatment. The standard manual and machine-based techniques when employed appropriately can be useful components of an injury treatment program; but in the case of serious, chronic injury they seem to be limited in their capacity to specifically and directly effect longer-lasting, thorough benefit for the whole spectrum of processes and tissue changes described in Chapter 5.

There are distinct differences from the standard treatment in my manual therapy model. The relation of the model to structural/functional changes of recovery will also be described in Chapter 5 and seen in the case studies. It utilizes more of a whole-body approach. This incorporates a greater degree of attention to overall and regional alignment patterns and reduction of muscular and fascial pulls on the injured tendon/ligament. In general, I do more work to normalize the joints near the injured structure. There are manual methods for the injured tissue and its fibers including normalization of fibrous alignment, which are unusually specific (e.g. BMC and Fascial Release). The specific fiber and tissue work seems to be in greater detail. This directly addresses the problem of laxity and weakened, stringy, thin fibers, which receives little direct manual attention in other approaches. Counterstrain, Zero Balancing, and BMC methods are able to reduce inappropriate proprioceptor activity in and around the tendon/ligament and normalize segmental dysfunction, more specifically than the standard approach.

In general, my approach incorporates extensive usage of indirect techniques and is less forceful than some of the manual procedures of the conventional model (e.g. cross-fiber massage), which actually work with the localized area of injury. This low-force approach is useful for avoidance of exacerbating inflammation, irritation, and damage that can occur with overtreatment (including exercise therapy) of structures that may be very fragile. Low-force work can successfully locate and address the neural and specific localized tissue anomalies and changes in small zones of a joint, ligament, or tendon (which can be small structures in total). This encourages an ongoing fine perception by the clinician during the treatment procedure, and thus can be more precise.

The therapeutic model I use includes a manual approach to a fine-tuning of the electromagnetic activity of the tissues (see "Techniques" section), which is not found in the standard approach. The electro-stim and T.E.N.S. unit do not appear to harmonize this activity in the same way. I also incorporate more attention through manual techniques to improving neural function of the ligament/tendon and its interconnections (including structural alignment patterns) locally and generally. As is illustrated in the case studies here, my model of manual therapy also differs from the standard medical model in that it incorporates the concept of a significant possibility for recovery from serious, chronic tendon/ligament injury with conservative care.

Personal Background and Training

This description of personal background is intended to illustrate development of the skills, capabilities, and techniques involved in this therapy model for tendon/ligament injuries. It shows the gradual interweaving of various interests and methods to form my particular therapeutic approach.

Entry into this field grew out of physical activities of the high school and college years including various sports (baseball, tennis, and track), yoga, and dance. This led to an interest in learning about the body's structure and function. The impetus to an active life led to six years of employment after college in carpentry and farming, and ongoing participation (to the present) in running, weight training, and cycling. My learning about body function has been enhanced by study of t'ai ch'i and ballet (with Brynar Mehl).

Entry into the field was also stimulated by my interests (in college at C.C.N.Y., and post-college years) in the study of anatomy, sensing the body in a meditative practice, and the study of Chinese medicine. I will start here with my interest in Chinese medicine, which in 1970 led to the study of acupressure therapy with Kazuko Yamasaki, who had been trained in Japan. My study with her in Chico, California evolved into an apprenticeship lasting four and a half years. In 1973, I started a part-time private practice. Along with the techniques and theory, what I learned from Mrs. Yamasaki was valuable orientation as to the attitudes, way of life, and ethical sense of a health practitioner. In 1974 and 1975 I trained in shiatsu with Shizuko Yamamoto at the East-West Institute in New York and received a Certification in Acupressure Therapy in 1975.

From learning and practicing acupressure I gained a familiarity with the interrelation of a complex web of the entire organism, and familiarity with a sense of the electromagnetic activity of the body—both of which are useful in dealing with tendon/ligament injury. Acupressure (including some reflexology) was a major part of my practice for the first five years.

Sensing the body with a meditative focus began during my participation in yoga and free-form dance during college and post-college years, and was also part of more formal meditation after college. The practice of sensing is the application of awareness (full, active attention) to the perception of the sensations of one's body, including the subtleties of the internal proprioceptive and kinesthetic sense. This encompasses the perception of internal rhythms (breath, pulse, etc.). My motivation here was curiosity and interest in the way the body functions and a desire to increase health and well-being. In the course of sensing I monitor body sensations and identify zones of tension or blockage, while allowing effortless, balanced motion of basic body rhythms (breath, blood flow) in those zones and their aligned, relaxed connection to adjacent areas and the whole body. Sensing evolved into an integral part of a comprehensive practice of ongoing moment-to-moment awareness that gradually became more and more central in my life; I have received expert guidance (1975 to 1990) from Lew Colburn, a former Jungian analyst who became an overall mentor to me. I learned from him that the body can be an instrument for reaching clear awareness and have continued to practice sensing up to the present. It has helped in the learning and application of the clinical methods.

Sensing the body along with the physical activities stimulated an interest in learning anatomy and kinesiology. I started independent study in 1970, which has been informed by the sensing practice, and utilized books, manuals, and journals. I began studying anatomy with Bonnie Bainbridge Cohen in 1974 (see below) and have continued learning this subject all along, finding it invaluable in my clinical work, and eventually teaching courses in it.

My interest in anatomy and kinesiology led me to begin studying with Bainbridge Cohen in 1974. In her teaching of experiential anatomy, cognitive learning is integrated with inner sensation, movement, sound, palpation, and imagery. The student gains an embodied understanding of the material, in part through direct (immediate) experience of his/her body. Body-Mind Centering includes the development of fine perceptions (of one's own body and that of others) such as the palpation of subtle tissue changes and detection of small shifts of movement quality that are so useful for manual therapy. There is study of each major body system, fluid, skeletal, organ, etc., and its interrelation with the others in regards to alignment and movement patterns.

Bainbridge Cohen also teaches focused, effective techniques for tendon and ligament treatment that I have integrated into therapy practice, and have encouraged my interest in treating these injuries. Studies with her in 1974 and 1975 (and then at intervals up to 1995) had significant influence in the development of a clinical approach, in the direction of a more structural focus utilizing the principles of kinesiology. I completed the school's Practitioner Certification in the process (1985). Her example and instruction led to confidence that I could contact and beneficially affect even minute body structures in myself and in clinical practice.

In 1975 I started a manual therapy practice in the Bay Area. In 1976 and 1977 this was combined with part-time work doing acupressure with the chiropractic patients of Dr. George Casey in his office, gaining familiarity with chiropractic theory and practice management. Starting in 1977, I have maintained a full-time practice.

My interest in structural therapy led me to begin study of a derivative version of Counterstrain Technique in 1977 with an English osteopath. This began my involvement with Osteopathic manual therapy. I became certified as an instructor of this Counterstrain derivative in 1979, and started teaching courses. At that time I discovered Dr. Lawrence Jones' writings about his origination of Counterstrain, studied his manuals, and later took courses with him. His technique became a cornerstone of my practice. It helped with: sensing self-corrective forces in the body, utilizing an understanding of spinal mechanics, and realizing the efficacy of very gentle manual pressures to change the body structure. Dr. Jones' clarity of intention, economy of effort, and sense of humor have been a model to me as a health practitioner.

Another very experienced clinician who has been a role model is the osteopath and acupuncturist Fritz Smith, with whom I studied Zero Balancing in 1981 and 1982. Learning his method has helped the integration of structural therapy with acupressure. Along with Dr. Smith's technical expertise, his integrity and unpretentious approach to working with the whole person helped to deepen the efficacy of my work.

The osteopathic perspective was opening up for me, and the next component was Cranial Osteopathy. In 1982 I undertook the independent study of cranial anatomy, mechanics, and of the therapeutic techniques. This project was aided through guidance from a visiting Belgian osteopath, and from Paul Boudakian, a dentist who had received osteopathic training in Dr. Frymann's cranial courses. Starting in 1983, I completed a series of cranial technique courses taught by John Upledger, D.O. During this period I also received instruction from Richard MacDonald, D.O. and Jerry Slattery, D.O., and subsequently from Muriel Chapman, D.O., who, at that point in her eighties, influenced my sense of professional focus with her skilled simplicity and consistent deep attunement in her work.

The study and practice of osteopathic cranial work provided a more extensive sense of working with the interrelation of the musculoskeletal structure and the central nervous system—and a tactile appreciation of subtle tissue change and of subtle movements and body rhythms (CRI). It also incorporates Fascial Release techniques. As with all the methods I employ it utilizes a focus on the reciprocal forces and the patterns of the body, combined with precise attention to localized centers of dysfunction and stress.

In 1986, I began the study of osteopathic Visceral Manipulation with Jean-Pierre Barral, D.O., and then completed a progression of courses he taught. I found that working with the organs and internal body forces has been very beneficial for musculoskeletal problems. Dr. Barral's methods (which I have studied all along, and also taught) incorporate highly detailed knowledge of anatomy. They also include refinement of techniques for locating the centers of reciprocal tension patterns of the body, which are often the sources of dysfunction. I have been influenced by the scrupulous quality of his research as well as his clinical precision and emphasis on accuracy founded on confidence in the perceptual capacity of the human hand.

In 1985 I sustained a serious injury to my left triceps tendon, largely due to overzealous weight lifting exercise. There was significant tearing and then wasting of the fibers, and I was forced to stop my therapy practice for two months and then resume work gradually. During this time and over the next seven years, I underwent a number of different treatments (both standard and complementary) in a cycle of partial healing and reinjury from working. The tendon was assessed as being permanently damaged by two orthopedists (1986 and 1989) who advised surgical treatment with hope of only partial recovery. In 1992 I finally achieved close to complete recovery of the health of the tendon (90 to 95 percent) through a combination of strategies I'd already used, including osteopathic treatment—augmented by some intensive treatment of skilled Fascial Release, combined with the structural insights of Weslynn Hants, a medical intuitive. I gained an enhanced ability to work with these injuries in clients, including a sense of tissue health, precise alignment of fibers, and electromagnetic condition. Good health of the triceps tendon has continued and improved up to the present.

A Master's degree in biomechanics from Antioch University completed in 1996 enabled me to broaden the scientific and theoretical background for clinical work. This encompassed a range of subjects from the more standard curriculum to relevant physics, architecture, and muscle physiology. Connective tissue and its repair mechanism was a major emphasis of the program.

My professional training has been enhanced by teaching trainings in osteopathic-derived structural therapy since 1979. These have been both independently organized courses, and courses through institutes such as: The School for Body-Mind Centering, The Upledger Institute (assisting with Dr. Barral's methods of Visceral Manipulation), Authentic Movement Institute, and Axelsson's Institute (Stockholm).

Professional training in manual therapy has been founded on following my interest, finding what is needed for successful results. This has led me to timely instruction from expert teachers, clinical practice, and ongoing independent study; the combination has enabled crafting of a therapy model consisting of a blend of techniques, aptitudes, and principles. Its active use will be seen in the case accounts that follow.

CHAPTER 4

Case Studies

The central focus of this chapter is the two in-depth case study reports from my clinical practice, supplemented by ten shorter case reports. The first section is a discussion of the research design utilized to carry out my investigation of the benefits of manual therapy for tendon and ligament injuries. The case studies are a key component of this design. The reader may want this perspective on the rationale for, and the mechanism and validity of this style of research, or go directly to the case reports.

Research Design and Methodology

My research includes a description and examination of the model of the therapeutic approach I am using (it combines several methods and certain skills), as it is employed in clinical situations, in order to determine its efficacy. The research data illustrates this therapeutic model and its usage. This data includes the presentation and analysis of case studies from my practice and also the relevant theory, scientific research findings, and other therapeutic model (standard medical) that have already been presented. The data involved in discussion of therapeutic and theoretical models is gathered from readings, interviews, and clinical experience.

A central component of this research study is the case studies. I use a protocol for the case study reports which Robert Yin calls linear-analytic and chronological.[89]

The data sources utilized in the case studies are:

- The thorough clinical notes I have taken during the course of treatment, which include the patients' reports of their condition, discussions with and reports from other clinicians who have treated the patient for the condition, plus all the varied clinical findings I have made.

- Medical diagnosis of the condition, partially derived from X-rays and MRI findings.

- Discussions with the patients subsequent to the end of the course of treatment.

The criteria of therapeutic efficacy (variables) that I use are:

- range of motion of the joint(s) adjacent to the injury;

- findings as to the quality of the affected tissues, i.e., resiliency, tone;

- patient's capacity to function using the affected area; and

- comfort/pain.

The case study research design allows the incorporation of phenomenological methods that can translate nonverbal, perceived forms into articulate and precise descriptions.[90] I use both qualitative and quantitative methods in assessing the above-mentioned criteria of effectiveness.

A demonstration of the clinical skills I have developed in my work is relevant in substantiating the validity of the research findings, and also in construction of the therapeutic model I am using; so included as research data is a description of my training and relevant parts of my background/experience. A substantial degree of the accuracy of the research findings and efficacy of the therapy depends on a certain level of perceptual skill, so I have described how this has been developed over the course of my career.

Essential elements of this design are discussion of the standard medical approach to the treatment of tendons and ligaments and some pertinent theory and scientific research data. This places in context the clinical work described in the case studies. It is a basis to construct a therapeutic model and to establish validity of my findings. The recent theory and scientific findings on the mechanism of connective tissue repair and healing are background for, and a component of, the therapeutic model that I am constructing.

I will now discuss how the data will be analyzed. The individual cases will be reported, and will be followed by a cross-case analysis in which significant features of the cases are compared and contrasted. Time-series analysis will be used at this point and in the individual case reports. This involves showing a progression over time of certain specific indicators (criteria) to establish causal relationships. Pattern matching is another form of analysis to be utilized. This method compares an empirically based pattern to a predicted one. Nonequivalent dependent variables are identified (i.e., resiliency of the connective tissue, range of motion of the joint) and matched to a predicted outcome of therapy to determine efficacy. If the patterns coincide, the results will strengthen the internal validity of the case study.

The research design is not intended to evaluate therapeutic efficacy through the use of statistical generalization (randomized sampling). However, another form of analysis I will use to determine efficacy is analytical generalization (Yin),[89] similar to analytical induction (Nachmias),[91] in which one generalizes a particular set of results (case study) to some broader theory/model. This uses replication logic, which implies that if one can replicate (reproduce) a similar finding by using the therapy model in other cases, it is a reliable one. This generalization has elements of a hypothetical/deductive approach, and will be combined with inductive analysis (Patton)[92] that begins with specific empirical observations and builds toward a general pattern. This "discovery mode" is similar to Glaser's and Strauss's grounded theory[93] approach to theory-building.

Some of the rationale for this research design has been made in the preceding paragraphs, but I will now focus specifically on this topic. Employing a case-study approach is appropriate when research is conducted in a real-life situation (i.e., my clinical practice) with a large number of variables and a context that cannot be tightly controlled. Because case studies examine people in or close to real situations and because they do not distort naturally occurring behavior through experimental manipulation and the creation of artificial conditions, they may offer better external validity than do controlled experiments.[89] Yin sees the case study approach as the preferred research strategy when "how" or "why" questions are being asked, both of which concern me in this situation.[89] In what Patton calls "purposeful sampling," certain cases are selected in order to find information-rich cases for study in depth.[92]

Further rationale for this design is that research with detailed cases affords the opportunity for a more thorough, in-depth investigation and understanding. I am using intensity sampling, where I have found excellent cases with some typical qualities (not extremes) that are of sufficient intensity to elucidate the phenomena of interest. My case selection also has elements of what Patton calls critical case sampling, in which a case makes a point quite dramatically "...if it (the therapy) works here, it can work in most instances."

I am a participant-observer in this research and while this has advantages, it makes it particularly important to strive for accuracy and to guard against bias. One benefit is that a participant-observer can discover things to which no one else has ever really paid attention, or had such good access. He can learn about things that subjects may be unwilling to discuss in an interview. It enables the evaluator to understand the context within which the program operates, and to access personal knowledge and direct experience as resources to aid in understanding and interpreting (Patton).[92]

Bias is a pitfall for any researcher, but the participant-observer must be particularly vigilant in watching for it. Here are some methods/

approaches that I use to minimize bias. One tactic is to give the sense that my analysis has taken into account all the available evidence and that my information-gathering is thorough. I report and focus on the most essential and significant aspects of the case study. It is helpful to build a chain of evidence (Miles and Huberman, Yin) that allows a reader to follow the derivation of evidence over time.[89,93]

The use of multiple sources of evidence minimizes bias and strengthens credibility, validity, and reliability. Using reports, medical diagnosis, letters, and patients' self-reports along with my own clinical findings that trace several variables is beneficial here. The use of multiple sources leads to triangulation in which converging lines of inquiry lead to the same conclusion, and thus strengthens credibility. In writing about case study research, Merriam describes methodological triangulation as the use of multiple methods of data collection (i.e., interviews, observations, physical evidence).[94] Bias is also minimized by comparison with the standard medical model (the predominant treatment mode in this society), thus adding perspective to my methods and analysis. Demonstrating my prior expert knowledge of the subject matter and clinical methods adds credence that my research is thorough, skilled, and relatively impartial.

In regard to the issue of bias as it relates to the professional (osteopathic) context in which much of this research is being done, it is assumed in my work that the professional integrity of the clinician would involve attempting to achieve the best result in any case (researched or not). So, the main issue as relates to bias would be accuracy and impartiality in assessment and reporting. Merriam says that one goal in case research is to have observations recorded systematically and with some detachment, a skill that I have practiced for a long time in recording clinical notes about clients. These notes are used extensively in the research.

Also in regard to bias and clarity, a potential pitfall for a participant-observer is to be so immersed that one is oblivious to the patterns in the situation (Patton, Yin). Both the osteopathic and Body-Mind

Centering methods that I practice are based on very rigorous, careful observation (assessment of oneself and others), and the recognition of patterns. This requires alertness and discipline—and a certain level of impartiality.

The skilled clinician learns to monitor (evaluate) the effects he is having on the subject both through his intervention and attitude, which can change in the course of treatment. He is, in effect, part of the data (which can be reported)—and the awareness of this is the skill of a good clinician, and of a good researcher. In this area, Patton asserts that conveying an understanding of the interaction between the evaluator and subject gives the study situational and interpersonal authenticity.[92] Discussion of the preceding factors illustrates how my professional skills and opportunities as a clinician are advantageous in the context of this research design and its implementation.

I am including studies of cases that are already completed. The response to concerns about this is that these are reports of thorough notes taken during the therapy and materials (e.g. MRI) that were done at that time. These were in-depth cases with systematic notes at each treatment session; I am not primarily relying on memories of past events. The cases are chosen because they are information-rich and very instructive. It is useful in employing post hoc studies that they be placed in context, such as how they fit into the overall population. Context is also established by discussing what factors are positive or negative indicators for success in the therapy (e.g. client's willingness) and how they obtained in these cases.

Case Study 1 (Janet C.)
History and Diagnostic Findings

Janet C., a forty-three-year-old university administrator, started treatment with me for problems with her right and left tendo-calcaneus. The right tendon was more problematic but she suffered from constant pain in both, and could walk only one block because of severe pain that resulted from any further walking. The subject reported that she had a high pain threshold, e.g. occasionally having dental fillings without anesthesia. The problem started one and a half years previous to this time. Janet said that her most severe pain occurred when attempting to walk after any interval of inactivity. This was most pronounced on awakening in the morning, when she experienced extreme stiffness of ankle movement for four or five minutes. The cause of the tendon injury was not apparent. Her office job involved mostly sitting.

She had consulted with an orthopedic surgeon and a podiatric surgeon specializing in sports medicine. An MRI showed the thickening of the right and left tendon sheaths and both nodules and defects in the right tendon. The right Achilles tendon sheath was thickened to three times its normal dimension. The podiatric surgeon said that he had only seen the level of severity of this type of serious Achilles tendon injury in marathon runners. Janet had a desk job and her primary form of exercise was walking. A test for rheumatoid arthritis proved negative. Her general health was good.

She had six weeks of physical therapy for the injury (three times weekly). This consisted of heat and cold applications, ultrasound, electro-stimulation, massage, whirlpool, and some stretching and strengthening exercises. There was also usage of heel lifts and longitudinal arch supports. There was no improvement from this treatment.

Previous to the physiotherapy, the orthopedist had prescribed various anti-inflammatory medications and administered bilateral cortisone injections. There was some relief but the effects disappeared within two weeks of completion.

During the whole period since the onset of the injury Janet had weekly sessions with a massage therapist, which also didn't appear to change the condition of the tendons. After physiotherapy she received treatment from a physician who administered acupuncture and homeopathic therapy.

Janet then consulted a podiatric surgeon whose examination revealed nodules and soft tissue masses in and around the tendons. His biomechanical evaluation revealed a modest pronation pattern. He found extreme limitation of movement, and administered injections of local anesthetic and homeopathic substances and a further course of anti-inflammatory medication. After a month, finding no appreciable improvement, he told Janet that he suspected some type of collagen disease and recommended surgery for both tendons to reduce the thickening of the tendon sheaths. She was advised that there was a possibility that the adhesions could return after surgery.

Janet was referred to me for treatment by her general practitioner and by the podiatrist, who suggested she try it for a month while he was away, with the prospect of surgery on his return. She was not very enthusiastic about the surgery, in part because there was confusion about the cause of the problem and a lack of assurance that the condition would not reoccur.

My initial examination confirmed the findings of the MRI report. I found extreme sensitivity to touch on both the right and left tendons with accompanying swelling and chronic inflammation. Her movements of the ankle areas were quite limited. I told Janet that the possibilities for recovery through the osteopathic therapy appeared to require probably six months, and possibly as much as eight or nine months of treatment. It seemed that her cooperation involving adequate rest, limitation of activity, and gradually increasing exercise would be essential for success. I suggested weekly treatments initially followed by less frequency as sufficient progress occurred. I would have a much clearer picture of the possibilities for success after three treatments. She said she wanted to avoid surgery, would cooperate with the resting and exercise, and was quite willing to begin treatment.

Course of Treatment

At the first session, Janet reported that she had continuous pain (most pronounced in the right leg) and could walk no more than one block before it became almost intolerable. Any dorsiflexion of her ankle was painful and its maximum range was 10 degrees. Active plantar flexion was painful, particularly after 20 degrees, and the toe raise was weak. I found that even the mildest touch of the actual tendon areas produced more pain. I found joint restrictions in the lower spine, knee, and the joints of both feet. There was swelling and inflammation of the tendon areas, which were notice-ably thickened. The right leg was most problematic, particularly at an area on the medial aspect, two inches proximal to the tendon insertion. The tendon fibers exhibited some twisting and considerable inter-fiber adhesion.

At this first session I did Counter-strain positionings to free restrictions of the lower spine and of the foot (particularly the tarsal bones). There was also some Fascial Release work and ligament work for the joints of the foot. Specific treatment for the Achilles tendons consisted of induction and also separation of the fibers perpendicular to their length, in order to free the fibroses and adhesions. This was done using very mild pressures because of the degree of tenderness.

Janet reported at the second session, one week later, that she had some extra soreness after the first treatment

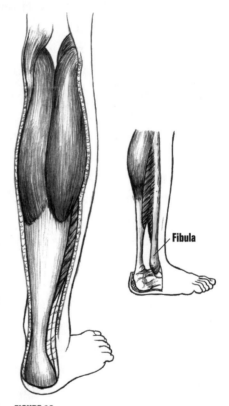

Fibula

FIGURE 19
Right Achilles tendon (tendo-calcaneus), posterior and lateral views. It is primarily a blend of the soleus and gastrocnemius muscle tendons and is the thickest and strongest tendon in the body.

that dissipated by the following day. I found that the left Achilles tendon was almost as sore to the touch as the right but not as problematic in terms of tissue irregularities or impaired mobility. The lower spine was somewhat more mobile. The electrical activity of the tendons had a jangled, uneven quality, and sense of "static." There were two noticeable areas of defect (tissue depression) in the right tendon: 1) a half inch from the calcaneal insertion on the lateral aspect 2) near the musculotendinous junction on the medial aspect. Each of these defects resulted from fibrous rupture of 35 to 40 percent of the total thickness of the tendon. I used some Visceral Manipulation techniques for freeing the lower abdominal/pelvic area. Fascial and Myofascial techniques were used to free restrictions and adhesions of the lower leg muscles and fascia including the tendon sheaths. There was pulsing in areas of the right tendon during the session, particularly during some induction methods.

At the third weekly session, Janet reported having slightly less pain upon awakening and noticed a little more flexibility. Walking was slightly easier although she was still not exercising. I found somewhat less edema and thickening of the right tendon and its sheath. With less overall swelling it became apparent that there was a spot on the medial side, two inches from the insertion, that was noticeably more thick and congested than its surroundings. The tendon fibers in general had a consistency that was brittle, stringy, and inelastic. As the right tendon was more problematic, reference from now on will be to this one except where otherwise noted. I worked with the knee joint and also with the proximal insertions of the calf muscles, using direct pressure on the Golgi tendon organs. There was also some use of techniques for freeing both ankle joints and the joints of the feet. It seemed particularly important to release fixation of the right cuboid bone. I used BMC techniques to improve the fluid movement through the tendon area (including mild pumping).

At the fourth session, two weeks later, Janet reported less stiffness and that the pain was no longer continuous. There was about one-third of the time when her legs were not painful. She was now walking three blocks at times, although this was still uncomfortable. I noticed less inflammation in both tendons and that the left side was less tender when palpated. Ankle dorsiflexion to 15 degrees was possible although still painful. We agreed that there had been some improvement of her condition and that it seemed worthwhile to continue the treatments at one-week (and occasional two-week) intervals. I did some work to normalize the electrical and magnetic activity of the tendon and its surroundings. There was application of techniques to realign the tendon fibers, mostly from Body-Mind Centering, with additional use of induction. I used some Visceral Manipulation methods in the abdominal area with particular attention to right kidney mobility.

The following week, the report was that there was pain about one-half of the time, with the exception of stressful activities such as extended periods of standing. The tendon sheath was less swollen and enlarged, and there were less adhesions (better mobility) between the sheath and the tendon. It was easier to work directly with the tendon because of the reduced tissue congestion of its surroundings. Janet's lower spine was freer, but still had some restrictions that were addressed with Counterstrain and Zero Balancing methods. I used these methods to work with the spine in all sessions throughout the course of therapy. Findings of excessive tension in both hamstring muscle groups led to treatment of their insertion areas and other methods for increasing their resting length.

Janet reported one week later, at her sixth treatment, that the upper (proximal) part of the tendon seemed less sore and that she had less stiffness on awakening. Her legs mainly hurt while walking, and she was now up to six blocks. She started exercising with toe raises. There was more elasticity of most of the tendon, and its fibers were better aligned. I continued to do specific work with the fibers by alternation of feeding in the ends of the tendon together and then separating them apart (I refer to the musculotendinous junction as one end of the tendon). Adjustments of the skeletal structure of the foot proceeded more easily, and the improvements of mobility and alignment were lasting longer.

The session after a two-week interval was focused particularly on the tissue congestion in the tendon and on its electrical activity. Janet

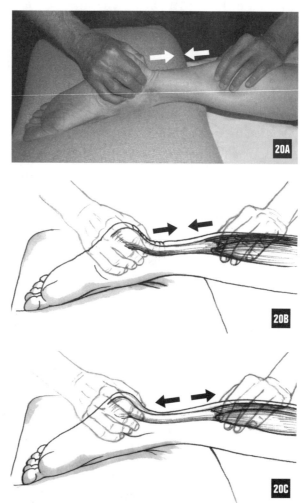

FIGURES 20A, 20B, AND 20C
The technique here is feeding in the ends of the Achilles tendon toward its center (20A, 20B), which can be alternated with drawing them apart (20C). This is directed toward realignment of its fibers and/or normalizing the tone and thickness of the tendon (see BMC techniques in Chapter 3). The tendon is placed here in a relaxed, slackened position with ankle plantarflexion; this is particularly helpful to the feeding in phase of the technique.

started to incorporate mild stretching exercise for the lower legs. Passive dorsiflexion up to 15 degrees was only slightly painful. There was less inflammation and swelling of the tendon. The two areas of defect in the tendon (see report of second session) were not as noticeable, as the tissues were starting to fill in there. The fibers in those areas had less weakness, "stringiness," and laxity. I found that pulsation of the tendon area during treatment occurred more readily and that the blood flow through the area felt more full and even.

My findings the next week were that active plantarflexion of her ankle was painful only after 40 degrees (50 degrees is full range).[84, 85, 86] Janet said that she experienced some soreness in her calf muscles during walking. There was some soreness in the ten-

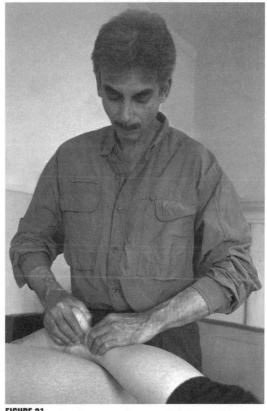

FIGURE 21
Normalizing the fascias deep to the Achilles tendon. These include the tendon sheath and the periosteum of the tibia and fibula.

dons proximal to her left knee. I did some work with both knee joints and with the tendons both proximal and distal to the knee. The techniques utilized for this were Counterstrain and direct fiber work with the knee area tendons. In addition, I applied Fascial Release methods to free fascia in and around the calf muscles. The area of congestion in the Achilles tendon two inches proximal to the insertion (see report of third session) was not as thick and had better elasticity. The tendon fiber alignment was closer to normal parallel arrangement.

Janet reported two and a half months from starting therapy that she had only minor pain on awakening and starting to move. She was walking up to ten blocks with some pain toward the latter part of the walk. She could now dorsiflex up to 20 degrees (full range) with the last 5 degrees being painful.[84, 85, 86] Her calf muscles were getting stronger from exercise, including the toe raises. I found soreness during palpation in her feet and calf muscles. There was some realignment work done for the bones of the foot. Both cuboid bones still seemed to be prone to fixation. It was much easier now to work under the tendon (next to the bone) because there was much less thickening of the tendon sheath and of the fascia deep to the tendon.

The therapy was progressing well enough for me to recommend that treatments once a month would be sufficient. At the tenth session Janet reported that she was now wearing three-quarter-inch heels comfortably, and was concerned that she still had discomfort when she wore flat shoes. She was doing more walking and her toe raises were stronger. I found that the hamstring muscles were tight, had limited movement range, and needed a longer resting length. The tissue quality of the Achilles tendon was better in its elasticity and tone. I did some work with its musculotendinous junction. There was usage of acupressure techniques for the foot and leg to improve the electrical activity. Some BMC and induction methods were used to improve articulation and movement between the tibia and fibula.

The following month, Janet said that she had only minor pain with a few everyday movements. She could now walk one mile and would have pain only in the latter half of this. She was doing more stretching. I found that her left leg needed more attention and increased my focus on it in this session. The excessive fluid accumulation was gone from the right tendon area. There was very little thickening except for the medial area two inches proximal to insertion. I continued to work with the anterior tibio-fibular area.

When I saw Janet the next month, she was able to wear shoes with half-inch heels with comfort. This was five and a half months from starting therapy. Walking one mile was no longer painful. Her ankles had complete range of motion (both active and passive) with only slight pain at the end of dorsiflexion. Her lower spinal and sacroiliac joints now had significantly less restriction. This was also the case for the lower abdominal and pelvic visceral structures. The electrical and magnetic activity of the tendons seemed relatively normal. The two previous major areas of defect in the tendon tissue were no longer present. As I had done in all the sessions, I worked with the alignment and mobility of the bones of the feet. There was also application of techniques to fine-tune the alignment and mobility of the tendon fibers and their bundles. Regular therapy was no longer necessary, and I suggested to Janet that she keep me informed of her progress and call if there was any problem.

At a follow-up session five months later, Janet reported that she had been doing more walking, occasionally up to two miles. The only occurrence of mild pain was at the end of a longer walk. She had complete pain-free range of motion in the ankle joints and was quite comfortable wearing half-inch heels. I found some slight thickening of two places in the right tendon. Janet felt this may have been caused by some increased exercise on a recent vacation. I did some work to thin out these adhesions and found that the tendon tissue normalized quite easily.

Follow-up and Comments

Janet was a cooperative client in her willingness to adjust her activity levels as recommended. She rested her legs and did walking, stretching, and strengthening exercises in accordance with my advice. Her attitude was good considering the discomfort she experienced, and she became increasingly optimistic as the course of treatment progressed.

After Janet's treatment was completed, the podiatric surgeon referred other patients with Achilles tendon problems to me. Janet reported to me that after an examination in the latter stages of my therapy with her, he remarked, "He did this with his hands?" When I saw him at a meeting two years later, he said good-naturedly, "You cost me a surgery."

One year after my last treatment, Janet was seen for another condition by the physician who had treated her tendon condition with acupuncture and homeopathy. She also had a session with a chiropractor she had seen in the early stage of the tendon injury. The Achilles tendons were examined by both of these practitioners. They remarked on a major difference in the tendon condition—noticing the healthier tissue quality, lack of swelling and inflammation, and normal range of motion and function of the ankle joints. These changes had also been noticed by the podiatric surgeon in a follow-up examination.

When I interviewed her two years later, Janet reported that she had been surprised that the tendons recovered so quickly during my therapy with her. She has continued to be pain-free and her tendons have not caused her any limitation of walking distance since that time. She is able to go barefoot while walking in her house, and to comfortably wear shoes that have only one-third- to quarter-inch heels.

Case 1 Progression (Janet C.): (Right Achilles Tendon)

PROGRESS	COMFORT/PAIN	CLINICAL FINDINGS/ TISSUE QUALITY	RANGE OF MOTION (PAIN-FREE)	FUNCTION	THERAPEUTIC TREATMENT/RESPONSE
begin therapy	- pain is continuous; worst in a.m., on arising, and after any inactivity (right leg worst, but left leg also quite sore)	- more pain on slightest touch - low back (spine) restricted - S.I. joints tight - knee joints tight - joints of arch tight - tendon is thickened, inflamed - area 2 inch proximal to lower insertion (medial) is worst - fibers twisted, stuck together	- any dorsiflexion from neutral is more painful, can't go more than 10° - wears heels - doesn't stretch anymore	- weakness of toe raise - any walking very painful - can walk one block before almost intolerable	- assessment - work with spine - work with foot, especially tarsal bones - work with tendon, painful, thinning out adhesions around it
1 week (from start)		- electrical, sense of "static," jangled - two areas of defect in tendon: ½ inch proximal to insertion (lateral side), and 4 inch proximal to insertion (medial side) - left leg almost as sore to touch - lower spine slightly looser	- active plantarflexion is painful, particularly after 20° - normal maximum range-passive is 20° dorsiflexion, 50° plantarflexion		- sore after session, but this dissipated by next day - Fascial Release for leg muscles - some pulsing in areas of right tendon during induction, then subsided - work with lower abdomen
2 weeks	- slightly less pain in a.m. than before	- spot on medial side, 2 inch from insertion, has major disruption of fibers - slightly less thickening of tendon sheath - slightly less swelling - consistency of fibers is stringy, brittle, inelastic	- more flexible in a.m. - dorsiflexion (slight) passive, is not quite as painful	- walking slightly easier - still not exercising	- work with knee joint, proximal insertions of calf muscles - techniques to improve fluid activity in tendon - work with foot (realignment of ankle joint, cuboid fixated)
4 weeks	- pain is now not continuous, some periods not painful (about one third of time)	- seems less inflamed - left leg tendon is less tender to touch	- notices less stiffness in a.m. or after inactivity - 15° dorsiflexion possible, still painful	- walking three blocks, some pain - localized stretching still quite painful	- work to realign tendon fibers - left leg responds well, pulsation during treatment - visceral work, right kidney

Case 1 Progression (Janet C.): (Right Achilles Tendon)

PROGRESS	COMFORT/PAIN	CLINICAL FINDINGS/ TISSUE QUALITY	RANGE OF MOTION (PAIN-FREE)	FUNCTION	THERAPEUTIC TREATMENT/RESPONSE
5 weeks (from start)	- pain now half of the time	- lower abdomen not as tight - spine is freer - hamstrings tight - sheath is thinner - adhesions are less between sheath and tendon			- work on hamstrings, insertions - can work more easily on tendon because less adhesions around it - work with lower spine (done in all sessions)
6 weeks	- upper part of tendon "seems more sore"	- tendon fibers have better alignment - better elasticity of most of tendon	- continues to have less stiffness in a.m.	- legs now hurt mainly when walking - walking six blocks, some pain - starts toes raises	- adjustments of foot skeletal structure are holding longer, easier response - work with attachment of tendon on calcaneus
8 weeks	- legs mainly hurt when walking	- electrical pattern of tendon seems more even - less swelling, inflammation - two areas of defect not as noticeable, starting to fill in, fibers not as lax	- passive dorsiflexion to 15° only slightly painful	- calf muscles weak - start mild stretching of calf muscles	- pulsation of tendon areas happens more readily—blood flow feels more complete - continuation of work to reduce congestion in the tendon
9 weeks		- soreness proximal to left knee in tendons - spot 2 inches proximal to insertion is not as thick, more elastic	- active plantarflexion is only painful after 40°	- soreness in calf muscles when walking	- work with knee joint tendons proximal, distal to knee - fascia around calf muscles - alignment of tendon fibers is more normal - work more easily under tendon (next to bone)

Case 1 Progression (Janet C.): (Right Achilles Tendon)

PROGRESS	COMFORT/PAIN	CLINICAL FINDINGS/TISSUE QUALITY	RANGE OF MOTION (PAIN-FREE)	FUNCTION	THERAPEUTIC TREATMENT/RESPONSE
10 weeks (2½ months)	- only minor pain when awakening and moving	- feet sore, medial calf muscles sore - significantly less thickening of sheath and fascia under tendon (next to bone)	- can dorsiflex to 20°, last 5° is painful	- toe raises starting to strengthen - walks ten blocks, some pain	- realignment of bones of foot, cuboid still gets fixated
14 weeks	- concerned with discomfort wearing flat shoes (is wearing ¾ inch heels)	- tight hamstrings - tissue quality of tendon is better	- limited range (hamstrings)	- doing more walking - toe raises stronger	- more work with musculo-tendinous junction - work to articulate free movement of tibia from fibula - acupressure techniques
18 weeks	- little pain with movements	- left leg needs work - swelling of right tendon is gone, thickening almost completely gone except for spot 2 inches proximal to insertion		- walk one mile; pain only in latter half - doing more stretching	- more work with anterior tibio-fibular area - more work with left leg
22 weeks (5 months)	- can wear shoes with ½ inch heel	- electrical, magnetic qualities seem normal - areas of defect not present	- complete (active, passive) range of motion - very slight pain at end of dorsiflexion	- walk one mile without discomfort	- continue work with bones of foot (this being done in all sessions) - work with inter-fiber mobility
10 months (follow-up)	- slight pain with longer walks	- follow-up - slight thickening returns after much more activity - tissue quality is healthy	- complete range of motion - can now comfortably wear shoes with only ½ inch heel	- has been walking more, occasional two mile walks	- thinning out fascia, responds well

Case Study 2 (Robert H.)
History and Diagnostic Findings

Robert H., a forty-eight-year-old physical therapist, initially sought treatment from me for an injury to the ulnar collateral ligament of the metacarpophalangeal (MP) joint of his right thumb. Future references to "the ligament" in the case account are to this structure. Although the injury had occurred over six months before, he described his condition as very little improved, despite having had consistent treatment for it. The ligament was injured when he caught his thumb on the edge of a heavy table that was falling as he was moving some furniture. There was a sudden forceful stretch of his thumb away from his palm (lateralwards, and somewhat anterior).

Two weeks after the injury, he consulted an orthopedic surgeon (who did much of his practice with hand problems) who found a serious sprain of the ligament, estimating that 55 to 60 percent of its fibers were torn. An MRI had shown the tears of the ligament fibers and some damage to the postero-medial part of the MP joint capsule. The orthopedist found laxity of the ligament, inflammation and effusion of the joint, and a strain of the extensor tendons of the thumb. Compression and distraction elicited pain of the ligament and joint, as did flexion and any lateralwards pressure. Robert was given an option of surgical repair, which he declined, and was referred to physical therapy. My reports of the sessions with the orthopedist at this time (also five months later and during my treatment) are from the medical records and Robert's account.

Robert had started physical therapy one week after the injury, and the therapist's report at that time described swelling and inflammation of the joint and ligament. There was continuous aching of the area. There was pain with all the movement directions, as described above by the orthopedic surgeon. He found laxity of the ligament and evidence of a partial tear. Robert had ten sessions of physical therapy over a two and a half month period. The treatment was cold and heat, some electrical stimulation, ultrasound, massage of the hand muscles, and use of exercise and splints. Robert took a course of nonsteroidal anti-inflammatory medication for six weeks, and then at intervals after that.

Robert had returned to work two weeks after the injury, and found only minor improvement from the physical therapy. After that was completed he started treatment with a chiropractor who specializes in sports injuries. He had seven weekly treatments. The chiropractor's report at the last session describes thickening and stiffness of the ligament, along with laxity. He reports modest improvement during the initial treatments, then a plateau, and notes a tendency for reinjury from activity.

Robert was working half time, after being off work for one and a half weeks initially. He was doing one to two and a half hours of manual therapy daily (with some splinting of his thumb) and continued to feel pain and weakness with pressure and gripping with his right hand. Five months after the injury, he again saw the orthopedic surgeon, who found excess fluid in the MP joint along with inflammation. The ligament fibers still had some tearing, as well as thickening and scar tissue. There was still pain with compression, distraction, flexion of the MP joint, and abduction of the carpo-metacarpal joint. There was still strain of the extensor tendons of the thumb although somewhat less than in his first diagnosis. There was considerable laxity of the ligament. He recommended a repair surgery, and when Robert declined this he prescribed another course of physical therapy. The surgeon predicted that the surgery would strengthen the ligament and improve its functionality, but could possibly lead to ongoing adhesions and a problem with the MP joint.

There were five more physical therapy sessions with the same therapist over the next month. The report at the end of this sequence described essentially the same features as the orthopedist's last report. The MP joint and ligament were capable of very little motion without pain. It was reported that Robert was now getting only minimal response to treatment. There was a continuous aching in the ulnar collateral ligament/MP joint area. The anti-inflammatories reduced this somewhat, but there was no residual benefit when he stopped them. Robert had a setback from working shortly after this, and then started treatment with me.

Course of Treatment

At my initial examination I found Robert to be congenial, yet quite discouraged about the condition of his hand and his restricted usage of it. He did not want to have surgery but was considering it if his condition did not improve. At this point he was working half-time, was doing only one hour or less per day of manual therapy, and was avoiding handwriting as much as possible. Robert said that he had had some initial encouragement from his beginning treatments of the physical therapy and the chiropractic, but that the progress was not sustained. He found that whatever gains he made were easily reversed. There was constant aching of the ligament and the first MP joint.

Compression and distraction of the MP joint were painful. Any flexion of the MP joint was painful for the ligament, as was any of its medial axial rotation combined with abduction at the CM joint. There was some swelling of the joint area, particularly postero-medially. There was weakness and laxity of the ligament. Even very light touch of the joint/ligament elicited pain. The ligament had areas of stiffness and thickening and fibers adhering to each other, while some areas felt weak and overstretched. I felt one area in particular (closer to the proximal attachment) in which the fibers had poor continuity—they hadn't healed from the tear. The ligament fibers were not in parallel alignment and there were areas that felt "frayed." There was restriction and stiffness of the inter-carpal, carpo-metacarpal and radio-carpal joint areas, and a number of the intrinsic and extrinsic thumb muscles. The joints of the upper limb had significant restriction along with the fascia in the forearm and wrist. There were also restrictions in the cervical and upper thoracic spine, thoracic outlet, and thoracic and upper abdominal viscera.

I felt that the overall structural problems could benefit from osteo-pathic techniques, which would reduce excess stress on the ligament; there was significant potential for benefit from specific manual therapy work on the ligament and thumb. My sense was that recovery for the ligament would require consistent treatment along with conservative usage and exercise, and that if Robert was to proceed with my therapy, that he might achieve a substantial gain in functional usage of it in three months—and hopefully close to complete recovery of function in six to nine months. I suggested three treatments (one a week) to start, to see if there was good enough response to warrant continuing the therapy. He was receptive to trying the therapy and agreed to moderate his activity with his right hand and do exercise as suggested. I felt that he had some useful exercise strategies already and that two of the splinting devices he had could be helpful.

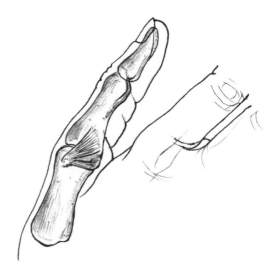

FIGURE 22
Ulnar collateral ligament of metatacarpophalangeal (MP) joint of thumb. The portion of the ligament that attaches on the first phalanx is more substantial than the portion attaching on the small sesamoid bone at the anterior (palmar) joint margin. Figure 13 (in Chapter 3) illustrates a therapy technique for this ligament.

At that initial session, I started some therapeutic techniques that I was to continue throughout the course of treatment. These were: clearing and thinning adhesions in the right ulnar collateral ligament of the first MP joint, and "feeding in" both ends of the lig-ament toward its center to encourage its knitting together. Both of these were done in combination with use of Counterstrain positioning for the medial part of the MP joint, which placed the ligament in the position of minimal stress (slackened). This had the immediate effect of increasing the fluid movement through the area, decreasing the swelling, and lowering the level of overexcitation of the localized tissue. I also did some Counterstrain techniques for restrictions of joints of the right wrist and CM joint of the thumb, and Counterstrain and Zero Balancing techniques for several of the cervical and thoracic spinal joints. In general the response was good.

I saw Robert for three more sessions at one-week intervals before decreasing the frequency to two-week intervals. At the second session I initiated some Fascial Release work to loosen rather stubborn tensions in the muscles of the right thumb, particularly the opponens pollicis, adductor pollicis, and the thumb extensors. There was some treatment for the cranial base and AO joint areas to encourage the balance and freedom of the entire spine and the dural membrane system. I did induction techniques for the thumb ligament and direct work with alignment of the ligament fibers where they were out of the normal parallel arrangement. The induction technique was directed particularly to an area of the ligament where there was still evidence of a tear (discontinuity of some fibers). This was about one-third of its distance from the attachment on the end of the first metacarpal bone. The response was some relaxation of the ligament (and its surrounding tissue) and a localized pulsation in the ligament area lasting about two minutes. Robert started some stretching at home for the forearm and wrist areas, and continued a moderate practice of some shoulder/neck and back stretches. He also did regular (three to five times per week) walking or stationary bicycling, which I encouraged him to continue.

The following week I found that mild compression of the MP joint was not as painful, and that he could do 5 degree to 10 degree slow flexion of the joint without pain in the ligament. He said that he was a little more comfortable on awakening in the morning, and that he found it somewhat easier to use the right thumb in his work of manual therapy. He was still using the thumb splint for this activity and was very cautious about using any thumb pressures. In this session I did some work to free restrictions of the upper abdominal organs and the pleura. I also worked with the thoracic outlet, and elbow and carpal joints. I worked to normalize the electrical quality of the ligament, in which I found a feeling of agitation and static. This resulted in a sense of more harmonious electrical activity in the localized tissues. The inflammation of the ligament and MP joint was somewhat reduced. Robert felt that he was getting some good result from the treatments. I agreed, and we decided to continue them.

At the fourth session, Robert said that handwriting was a little more comfortable, and that he was doing one and a half hours a day of manual therapy, mostly without the thumb splint. Swelling was lessened, I found less thickening in areas of the ligament, and the fibers were less clumped (adhered) together. His pain-free range of motion was increased (see chart) in MP joint flexion and CM joint abduction. I did some more specific work with the thumb joints and the fascia and muscles of the right forearm. The area of the torn ligament fibers was knitting together somewhat. In this session and others I used BMC techniques (including mild pumping) to improve fluid movement through the ligament and its surroundings.

We went to two-week intervals, and at the fifth session the ligament was less sensitive to touch. Robert said that it felt noticeably better after rest and particularly after two days of weekend rest (previously there was little or no improved comfort after rest). The inflammation was much lessened and the electromagnetic quality of the tissue more harmonious. I continued work with the cervical spine and cranial structure, using osteopathic cranial techniques. The cervical spine had better mobility but still was remaining restricted at the lower levels of C6 to T1. I did more work with the ligament fibers for their alignment, which was gradually improving. The small deposits I had found in the MP joint were reduced. He started resistance work with exercise putty for thumb and hand strengthening, which he had tried previously but was forced to discontinue because of pain. He was able to do some mild thumb pressure combined with medial axial rotation of the MP joint that was pain-free.

At the following session Robert reported lower levels of pain in the ligament, but that it was generally still stiff and sore on awakening in the morning. It was sore after working but recovered more quickly. He was now doing up to two hours a day of manual therapy on many days, taking a break in the middle. He could now flex the MP joint to 15 degrees free of pain and abduct the first CM joint to 15 degrees without hurting the MP collateral ligament. I continued many of the techniques I have previously described and specifically focused on the right wrist, in which the carpal bone joints and carpo-metacarpal joints were now maintaining better alignment but still needed better mobility. I found somewhat more strength in the thumb area, and that the ligament fibers had more integrity. There was slightly less laxity of the ligament.

He had up to 20 degrees of pain-free flexion of the MP joint at the next treatment, which was two months from the start of therapy. The ligament had significantly less thickening, except in an area near the center of the previously torn fibers. Robert had increased his time of manual therapy and was able to use some moderate pressure (longitudinal compression) with his thumb in a neutral position without discomfort. I worked with the abdominal and thoracic viscera for mobility, and treated the thoracic outlet. My work with the ligament fibers was getting a more rapid response. They relaxed and realigned more readily and were less sensitive to touch. The result was more balanced magnetic pulls and a smooth electrical current.

At the following session I found that the ligament fibers were knitting together well, although there was still some laxity of the overall structure. There was no swelling of the area. The CM thumb joint still had some stiffness, and I did Counterstrain, induction, and specific tissue work with the joint, its capsule and ligaments. There were gains in joint mobility and localized tissue resiliency.

Three months from beginning therapy, Robert reported that the ligament pain was mostly after exertion, and that there was usually very little pain on waking. He was doing up to two and a half to three hours of manual therapy on some days. The MP joint pain-free range had increased to 30 degrees of flexion. He was able to abduct the first CM joint to 25 degrees without pain in the MP ligament and was using the thumb somewhat more while the CM joint was moderately abducted. The MP joint still had some restrictions and irritation of the postero-medial area of its capsule. It had almost no swelling and had some small deposits in it. I worked to ease pressures on the joint through induction and Counterstrain, and some fascial and muscle work near the joint. There was particular attention to the periosteum of the first digit and its interface with the ligament. The extensor tendons of the thumb were recovering nicely.

There was significant focus on the overall spinal and cranial structure at the next session (now a three-week interval). I had given some attention to specific restrictions and overall balance of the whole spine in all the sessions, and in this one used more extensive concentration on some lumbar, sacral, and cervical restrictions. The ligament fibers still had some stiffness although their alignment was good. I did some work to restore resiliency. The electrical and magnetic sense of the ligament responded more rapidly and a smooth, steady currenting appeared during the treatment.

Robert reported three weeks later that he had increased his manual therapy work to three and a half hours usage on some days, and had experienced a little more soreness in the last week. The thumb muscles had developed some more tension since the last treatment, and he said that he hadn't done as much of the

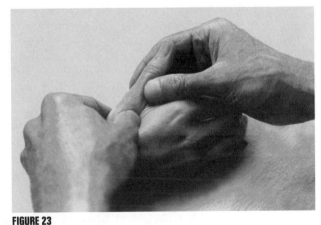

FIGURE 23
Counterstrain technique for MP joint of thumb. This positioning combines extension and adduction of the joint, and was used at several sessions. It places the ulnar collateral ligament in a relaxed state, which also facilitates other methods that were applied for its treatment.

moderate stretching and heat/cold and relaxation strategies recently. I did some work with the thumb muscles and forearm fascia and muscles, as we agreed that the increased tension had contributed to discomfort of the ligament. The muscle work included origin and insertion-point pressures, and Myofascial Release. He could flex the MP joint to 40 degrees without pain. The joint and ligament still had weakness, and I suggested he increase usage of the exercise putty for resistance work with the thumb and hand.

When I saw him next, the joint and overall ligament structure was stronger, including the localized tissue quality. There was some sense of electrical blockage in the ligament centered on the focal point of the previous tear. The work focused on increasing the integrity of the weak point in the ligament. I used techniques of feeding in the ends of the ligament toward center, alternated with very mild separations. There was also induction and focus on the normalization of electrical activity and magnetic pulls in this vulnerable zone. His carpal bone alignment and mobility were maintaining better condition and I continued to address this area.

At this time, the orthopedic surgeon examined Robert again. He found a great deal of overall improvement. There was no excess fluid in the MP joint. There was some laxity of the ligament. There was no pain from joint compression and slight pain from distraction. There was almost a normal range of pain-free motion (active and passive). He suggested that Robert continue his program, including more exercise for hand strengthening.

The last regularly scheduled session was three weeks later, five and a half months from starting therapy. I found that there was close to normal resiliency and elasticity of the ligament fibers. Robert reported that he felt pain usually only after a lot of usage and exertion, or if he stretched the ligament to extremes of its range while using thumb pressure. He worked full-time and was doing up to four and a half hours of manual therapy on some days, and in general doing as much as previous to his injury. He had 45 degrees of pain-free flexion of the

MP joint. I did some work with the fascia and muscles of the forearm. Also there was work with the much improved weak point of the ligament, and some fine-tuning of the fiber alignment. His cervical spine and thoracic outlet area were maintaining much better condition.

We made another appointment for six weeks that Robert had to cancel, and I then suggested that since he was feeling so good we could put off another session for a while unless he got into discomfort. I emphasized his keeping the hand and forearm muscles relaxed, particularly after days when he worked a lot.

Five months after his last treatment, Robert contacted me for a follow-up session to check his condition and do some fine-tuning. He reported that he was virtually pain-free in the ligament area. He was pain-free in the normal range of movement; 55 degrees of first MP joint flexion and 40 to 45 degrees CM joint abduction didn't bother the ligament.[95, 96, 97] He was working full-time, which was no problem as long as he monitored the hand and thumb muscles to make sure they didn't retain excessive tension. I found very little laxity of the ligament (about 5 to 7 percent). The ligament fibers had no thickening or adhesions except very slightly in the focal point of the injury. His overall upper body structure was in good condition. I did some spinal work and specific work with the ligament fibers to continue to improve the integrity in that focal point area. The overall resiliency of the MP joint and ligament was very good, as was the strength of the thumb and hand.

Follow-up

Robert was examined again by the orthopedic surgeon three months after our follow-up session, and soon after also had an informal assessment from the physical therapist who had treated him. The differences they noticed in the ulnar collateral ligament were: lack of swelling and inflammation, normal pain-free range of motion of the first MP and CM joints, and a general healthy tissue quality and normal tone (almost no laxity) of the ligament.

I spoke with Robert one and a half years later. He was working full-time and was able to do as much manual therapy as previous to his injury. Handwriting and computer usage was no problem at all. He said that his usage of his right hand was fully normal. His positive experience with Counterstrain technique has led him to study and start to incorporate it into his practice. He said that although my treatments had been somewhat unfamiliar to him at first, he had been willing to continue them when he saw consistent improvement. His comparison with the other therapies he had tried was that they were less specific in their approach to the injured ligament, less comprehensive in overall structural approach, and at times caused more irritation. The ligament had even less laxity now (less than 5 percent).

I found Robert to be quite cooperative as a client. He was highly motivated to recover and regain use of his hand to return to regular work capacity. Robert moderated use of his hand and followed an exercise regime with consistency and intelligence. He had been surprised at first that he was getting as much benefit from the treatment, but as it progressed he increasingly had the sense that his thumb could fully recover.

Case 2 Progression (Robert H.): Ulnar Collateral Ligament of First MP Joint (right)

PROGRESS	COMFORT/PAIN	CLINICAL FINDINGS/TISSUE QUALITY	RANGE OF MOTION (PAIN-FREE)	FUNCTION	THERAPEUTIC TREATMENT/RESPONSE
begin therapy	- constant aching that is increased from usage	ligament of MP joint: - adhesions in ulnar collateral ligament (areas of thickening) - some laxity of ligament - swelling, inflammation of MP joint - inflammation of ligament - feeling of electrical static - restrictions of carpal joints and some areas of cervical, thoracic spine	- any flexion of MP joint is painful - any medial axial rotation with CM joint abduction is painful for the ligament (active and passive)	- handwriting is painful to MP joint and ligament - pressure with end of thumb causes pain (compression) - using thumb to grip is painful, weak - working one hour a day of manual therapy is painful; works using splint for thumb	- assessment - work with clearing, thinning adhesions in ligament - Counterstrain techniques for joints of thumb and wrist - work with cervical, thoracic spine (Counterstrain) - "feeding in" both ends of the ligament toward center combined with Counterstrain for MP joint
1 week (from start)	- pain is most noticeable at postero-medial part of MP joint	- tension in thumb muscles, opponens pollicis, adductor pollicis, extensors - fascial and muscular tensions in forearm - some areas of ligament seem "frayed," torn - swelling, inflammation is most noticeable at postero-medial part of joint	- capable of mild hyperextension of MP joint, which is painful	- sense of weakness and pain of ligament, MP joint with axial rotation (medial) and abduction of CM joint - stretching for forearm, wrist	- work with thumb muscles - induction techniques for ligament - work with alignment of ligament fibers—led to some relaxation, pulsing of ligament and MP joint - work with AO joint, cranial bones, freedom of occipital and temporal areas of skull
2 weeks	- easier to find some comfort after heat/cold	- small deposits in MP joint - restrictions of mobility of upper abdominal organs - inflammation is slightly reduced - alignment of fibers shows some (more parallel) improvement	- mild compression not as painful - first 5° to10° of flexion all right if done slowly	- somewhat easier usage of thumb in manual therapy (uses braces/splint) - stretching for moderate extension of CM joint	- work to improve mobility of upper abdominal organs - elbow and carpal joints - work with forearm, thumb fascia, muscles - direct work with ligament - work with extensor tendons of thumb - techniques (BMC) to improve fluid movement through ligament area

Case 2 Progression (Robert H.): Ulnar Collateral Ligament of First MP Joint (right)

PROGRESS	COMFORT/PAIN	CLINICAL FINDINGS/ TISSUE QUALITY	RANGE OF MOTION (PAIN-FREE)	FUNCTION	THERAPEUTIC TREATMENT/RESPONSE
3 weeks (from start)	- ligament quality is now feeling better after rest - noticeably better after weekends - slightly less sensitive to touch in general	- swelling is lessened (of MP joint) - areas of thickening in ligament somewhat reduced (lessened) - fibers much less adhered together - area of tear in ligament is knitting together	- more tolerance for CM joint abduction, MP distraction still painful - 10° flexion all right (not painful)	- handwriting somewhat less problematic - working 1 hour/day manual therapy, not as painful - now doing 1½ hours; some days, 2 hours - now works without thumb splint	- work with CM joint of thumb - work with thumb muscles, extensor tendons - cervical spine and cranial structure - work with ligaments, results in more harmonious electrical and magnetic sense of the tissue
5 weeks	- electrical quality of ligament tissue is more harmonious - cervical spine is somewhat restricted, but has better mobility than before - deposits in joint are reduced - inflammation is much less	- starting to do medial axial rotation with power putty (pressing), not painful if done gently	- reports feeling more optimistic about possibility of recovery - continues to work with whole joint capsule - alignment of ligament fibers - work with fascia, muscles of forearm - work with thoracic outlet, mobility of pleura		- start exercise of small circles with thumb - most days, 1½ to 2 hours manual therapy - start power putty exercise; had done this before, but had to stop because of pain
7 weeks	- ligament, joint still sore after working, but recovers more quickly - still some pain in a.m. on awakening (stiffness)	- somewhat more strength in thumb area - ligament has more integrity (slightly less laxity) - less tension in thumb muscles but still need relaxation - wrist (carpal bone joints) and CM joints are maintaining better alignment—still need better mobility	- 15° flexion not painful - 15° abduction of 1st CM joint not painful for collateral ligament	- now using thumb splint mostly for handwriting and difficult tasks - 2 hours/day manual therapy; after first hour, soaks thumb in warm water - icing at end of day	- work with wrist alignment, mobility - work with upper abdominal viscera - work with muscles of thumb - "feeding in" both ends of ligament toward center, alternate with stretching apart—combined with Counterstrain for MP joint

Case 2 Progression (Robert H.): Ulnar Collateral Ligament of First MP Joint (right)

PROGRESS	COMFORT/PAIN	CLINICAL FINDINGS/ TISSUE QUALITY	RANGE OF MOTION (PAIN-FREE)	FUNCTION	THERAPEUTIC TREATMENT/RESPONSE
9 weeks (from start)	- ligament is less sensitive to touch	- ligament has much less thickening, except in one area of previously torn fibers - no swelling of ligament, joint	- starts stretching of thumb in abduction at CM joint, flexion of MP joint - 20° abduction is pain-free	- still needs to loosen thumb muscles after working - 2½ hours/day manual therapy, able to use some pressure (compression) through thumb	- work with thoracic outlet area - work with upper abdominal organs for mobility
11 weeks	- very little pain in ligament on waking - longer intervals with no pain	- carpal joints maintaining good mobility, alignment - ligament fibers are knitting together well, yet still some laxity	- 25° flexion is pain-free - 20° abduction of 1st CM joint is pain-free for collateral ligament	- longitudinal pressure with thumb is all right if moderate, and thumb is close to neutral position	- work with CM joint of thumb—still has some stiffness, good response - use of Counterstrain positionings for CM joint and for the MP joint
13 weeks	- pain is mostly after exertion	- ligament fibers are mostly in good alignment - still some adhesions, but much less - 1st MP joint is free of swelling, still has some stiffness, and a few small deposits	- 30° flexion is pain-free, active and passive	- some days 2½ to 3 hours/day manual therapy - is able to use thumb somewhat more when CM joint is in abduction	- work with joint capsule of CM joint, has some irritation of capsule at postero-medial area near collateral ligament - freeing tensions in pleura and mediastinum
16 weeks	- progressively less pain for regular, moderate usage	- ligament fibers still a bit stiff in some portions, although there is still some laxity	- 35° flexion is pain-free - 30% abduction of 1st CM joint is pain-free for collateral ligament	- 3 to 3½ hours/day manual therapy - able to do most manual activities if not pressured or stretched at extremes of range	- restoring resiliency to stiff portions of ligament fibers - work with cervical, thoracic spine as well as lumbar and sacral

Case 2 Progression (Robert H.): Ulnar Collateral Ligament of First MP Joint (right)

PROGRESS	COMFORT/PAIN	CLINICAL FINDINGS/ TISSUE QUALITY	RANGE OF MOTION (PAIN-FREE)	FUNCTION	THERAPEUTIC TREATMENT/RESPONSE
19 weeks (from start)	- has gotten some more soreness in last week	- integrity of ligament fibers is better - muscles of thumb have gotten tight since last treatment - also, some forearm muscle tightness - joint and ligament still has some weakness	- 40° flexion is pain-free	- 3½ hours/day manual therapy on some days - handwriting not a problem if he takes enough breaks - still avoids very heavy pressure on thumb	- work with thumb muscles - work with fascia, muscles of forearm - work with ligament fibers in central area of tear; electrical quality still obstructed, responds well
22 weeks (5 months)	- occasional soreness after working, but not consistently - still some tendency to have blocked electrical, magnetic quality - joint and ligament is feeling stronger (tissue quality)	- integrity of ligament fibers is better - muscles of thumb have gotten tight since last treatment - also, some forearm muscle tightness - joint and ligament still has some weakness - strength of some thumb area muscles is greater than others, need to balance	- 35° to 40° abduction of CM joints pain-free for collateral ligament	- using power putty more vigorously to build hand strength	- work with AO joint area and cranial structure - work with carpal bone alignment, mobility - work with ligament fiber alignment - Counterstrain for the MP joint
5½ months	- pain is felt mostly after much exertion/usage and if he stretches ligament to extremes of range	- better resiliency, elasticity of ligament fibers, close to normal - carpal area is in good balance	- 45° flexion pain-free	- some days does 4½ hours manual therapy, which is the same as previous to injury - still some caution of usage at extremes of range of motion - back to full time work	- work with center of ligament - work with electrical, magnetic quality of fibers - Fascial Release for fascia and muscles of forearm
10 months (follow-up)	- in general, is pain-free	- very little laxity of ligament - even center of ligament has only a very slight area of thickness, adhesion - thoracic outlet, better mobility	- 55° flexion pain-free, which is normal - 40° to 45° CM joint abduction (normal), is pain-free for collateral ligament	- working full-time - must monitor hand muscles to make sure they don't retain tension	- direct work with ligament fibers - work with upper body joint mobility

Ten Capsule Case Study Reports

For these ten case studies I used the same procedures and research model that was employed for the two in-depth cases in the first section of this chapter. The reports here are done in less detail, and the reader may refer to the technique descriptions in Chapter 3 for more information on the manual therapy methods. These reports add breadth and scope for the topic, further illustrating the nature of tendon/ligament health and treatment—and the variety of clinical situations where my therapeutic model is applied. All of these cases involve serious and chronic ligament or tendon injury.

The case reports are:

A. **extensor tendon of forearm muscles at lateral elbow (Alan R.)**

B. **two wrist ligaments (ulnar collateral and pisohamate) (Linda A.)**

C. **medial collateral ligament of knee (Alicia T.)**

D. **conoid and trapezoid ligaments of medial shoulder area (Ray N.)**

E. **flexor tendon of forearm muscles at medial elbow (Felix C.)**

F. **Achilles tendon (Kay S.)**

G. **capsular ligament of spinal facet joint and spinal intertransverse ligament (David B.)**

H. **annular ligament of elbow (Felicia M.)**

I. **distal hamstring tendon (biceps femoris) (Julia L.)**

J. **hip joint ligaments (pubofemoral, iliofemoral) (Mary S.)**

A. Extensor Tendon of Forearm Muscles at Lateral Elbow

Alan R. is a 53-year-old sculptor, artist, and housepainter who consulted me for a one and a half year problem with his left arm. He first noticed discomfort after an incident of gripping and pulling to move some heavy cable. After two months of continued work the pain and stiffness increased despite his use of anti-inflammatories. Pain centered on the lateral epicondyle area of the elbow and spread into the forearm. He saw two orthopedists (one is a specialist in repetitive strain injury) who diagnosed an extensor tendinitis with substantial tearing. Alan limited his work and had various treatments including medication, physiotherapy, acupuncture, and chiropractic. There was occasional relief but no lasting improvement. Six months after the injury, one orthopedist suggested surgical repair of the tendon.

I found the tendon to be lax and weak, with misalignment of its fibers and significant adhesions. Supination and pronation were limited to about 70 percent of normal range and were painful after the halfway point of the motion range. Elbow extension was limited by 10 degrees. Elbow flexion was painful in the last one-third of the range. Alan's wrist extensor muscles were weak and wrist flexion provoked pain after 40 degrees.

At a series of four weekly sessions I addressed restrictions of his lower cervical spine, left thoracic outlet, left shoulder, upper thoracic spine, and costovertebral joints. I worked to improve limited mobility of the upper abdominal organs, particularly the splenic flexure of the colon. His carpal bone alignment and mobility needed improvement, as did restrictions of the interosseus membrane between the radius and ulna. Alan further limited his housepainting and more strenuous art tasks during this time.

During three bi-weekly sessions after that I continued to work with constrictions of the forearm near the elbow, including the periosteum of the proximal radius. Loosening tension of the lower biceps and brachialis muscles was also very helpful for the tendon. Full elbow extension returned and all movements were improving. I continued to use localized techniques to re-align the tendon fibers, free its adhesions, and promote better tonus and decreased laxity.

In ensuing monthly sessions, the tendon appeared stronger and less "mushy." Four months after our initial session Alan was working about half-time, with very little pain. He used therabands for arm exercise. He noticed better coordination and fluidity of his arm usage. His pain-free range of motion was normal except for the last 10o of wrist flexion. I continued to work with the wrist flexor muscles and carpal joints to lessen constrictions and excessive tension.

After nine months from the start of treatment, Alan was working full-time and completed a house-painting job that he had put off for a while. He was still careful with strenuous sculpting tasks and used his arm more in neutral positions when exerting much force. The tendon fibers had knit together well. The orthopedist examined Alan and found the area to be normal. We stopped the monthly sessions at that time and I did a "tune-up" session six months later, at which his arm was in good condition.

B. Two Wrist Ligaments
(Ulnar Collateral and Pisohamate)

Linda A. is a 51-year-old nurse who injured her right arm and wrist in a bicycle accident. She consulted me ten months later, after orthopedic evaluation involving X-rays and MRI diagnosed a severe sprain of her wrist (involving significant ligament damage in the medial carpal area). The pain and instability was more pronounced on the ulnar side and involved much of the distal forearm. Linda had chiropractic, acupuncture, and treatment at a hand clinic. There was some initial improvement with each method, but no obvious benefit after that.

The MRI pointed to damage of the ulnar collateral ligament of the wrist and the neighboring pisohamate ligament on the wrist's palmar side. My initial findings were of inflammation, laxity, and fibrous disruption of those two ligaments. There was a nodule in each ligament amidst weakened fibers, indicating a poorly healed tear. Active and passive motions of Linda's wrist in all three planes were painful.

I began treatment of joint compression and anteriority (misalignment) of all the carpal bones, particularly the triquetrum and lunate. At five weekly sessions I addressed fixations of Linda's right thoracic outlet, shoulder, and elbow joints—and a marked tendency to ulnar deviation of the wrist. Her wrist movements became easier, with extension remaining most problematic. Linda continued to wear a wrist brace while working. The puffiness around the wrist was ended at this point.

At five bi-weekly sessions I continued localized techniques to realign the fibers of the two ligaments, while working to increase their tone and substance. The nodules were reducing nicely. There was still some pain at the end ranges of pronation and supination but she had regained a full range of motion for both. Linda was able to increase her computer usage at work if she used good ergonomic principles, but she still limited this to one and a half hours a day. She benefited by switching to a car with an automatic transmission. During this period she was increasing mild exercise for the arm and hand. The occupational therapist at the hand clinic told her she no longer needed to be seen there.

We continued treatments at three-week intervals. I worked with some restrictions in the flexor retinaculum of the wrist and the forearm fascias. A painful zone of her cervical spine became fully comfortable, and there was better flexibility of the cranial base. Six months after the start of treatment Linda had a full range of wrist extension and felt only a slight ache at the end of the range. She was still careful to use her arm and hand closer to neutral position when exerting much force. The tone of the pisohamate and ulnar collateral ligaments was close to normal.

Ten months after the start of treatment the ligaments had almost no laxity (about 5 percent) and Linda had regained full usage and mobility of her arm and hand. At a follow-up session the next year, the condition of the ligaments continued to be very good and the region free of pain.

C. Medial Collateral Ligament of Knee

Alicia T. is a 37-year-old psychotherapist who had a serious injury of the medial collateral ligament of her right knee resulting from a fall while running on a hilly trail. MRI findings in evaluation by an orthopedist resulted in a diagnosis of a Grade III injury (substantial tearing, instability) to the ligament along with a moderate injury of the medial meniscus. After an initial period using a crutch, she continued to use a brace cast to immobilize the knee due to its instability. Alicia then had physiotherapy and acupuncture.

She consulted me ten months after the injury because she still had substantial knee pain and disability, and had seen little progress for several months. The knee was still unstable with motions such as turning to the opposite side. I worked to reduce swelling of Alicia's knee area and generalized irritation of the knee joint capsule. At five weekly sessions I focused on improving the alignment of the joint and increasing and balancing glide of the patella. There was some atrophy of the quadriceps, particularly its VMO portion. I treated the collateral ligament for zones of thickening, weakened "stringy" fibers, and fibrous misalignment. The inflammation of the ligament and the meniscus started to subside.

On my recommendation Alicia started Pilates exercise with an expert trainer. She had undergone surgery for endometriosis two years previously, and had developed low back pain afterward. I used visceral manipulation techniques to reduce abdominal and pelvic adhesions that were restricting the ascending colon, duodenum, and liver. The fixations in the trunk initiated pulls and force lines through the entire right leg, causing extra strain on the knee. Freeing these fixations was helpful to the leg.

At four bi-weekly sessions I addressed fixations of her lumbar, sacroiliac, foot, and ankle joints. Fascial Release techniques for the quadriceps, other leg muscles, and fascias further balanced the tissue pulls through the knee area, reducing stress on the collateral ligament. Three months after the start of treatment Alicia could walk one mile comfortably on flat surfaces.

We continued sessions at three week intervals and the motion tests of her knee (anterior glide, tibial rotation) were much closer to normal.

This was five and a half months after starting treatment. I was still treating the collateral ligament for a zone with some thickening and adhesion, but the ligament had regained 90 to 95 percent of its normal substance and tone.

Eight months after the start of treatment, the orthopedic surgeon found almost no laxity of the knee and said that the meniscus seemed to be fully healed. Alicia was comfortably walking up to two miles with some hills, and bicycling several times a week for up to one and a quarter hours. When I checked the knee six months afterward, the collateral ligament had only 5 percent laxity. Alicia said that she had resumed jogging and was pain free.

D. Conoid and Trapezoid Ligaments of Medial Shoulder

Ray N. is a 48-year-old industrial mechanic who injured his right shoulder falling onto the arm in a motorcycle accident. When I first saw him nine months afterward, he was working on a limited basis with pain and limitation in the shoulder area. Evaluation by an orthopedic surgeon pointed to acromioclavicular joint dislocation as the most serious component of the injury. He had five months of physiotherapy and received ongoing massage therapy. Range of motion of Ray's shoulder had increased somewhat, but the pain, weakness, and stiffness hadn't improved for two months. Another orthopedist offered the option of surgery to correct instability of the AC joint involving a Grade III injury of the conoid and trapezoid (coracoclavicular) ligaments—which are integral to the joint's stability.

When I first assessed Ray's shoulder situation I found his most problematic directions of (active) movement to be: abduction limited to 65 degrees with pain after 40 degrees, external rotation limited to 60 degrees with pain after 40 degrees, and extension limited to 35 degrees with pain after 25 degrees. There was inflammation of the major bursae of the shoulder and restriction due to fibrosity of the glenohumeral joint capsule. The conoid and trapezoid ligaments were still inflamed, with the trapezoid in worse condition, involving more discontinuity of its torn fibers. At four initial weekly sessions I used induction techniques to improve fibrous alignment in the ligaments and encourage knitting together of weakened portions. I began working to reduce adhesions of the shoulder joint capsule and to ease strain of the rotator cuff muscles and tendons. Counterstrain positionings helped to free fixations of the shoulder, upper thoracic spine and ribcage, and lower cervical spine.

Ray still did most of his work with his left hand, but his right shoulder mobility was improving nicely. At three bi-weekly sessions I addressed restrictions of his cranial base, upper pleura and its attachments, and all thoracic outlet structures including the subclavius muscle and sternoclavicular joint. Compressions of the wrist and elbow joints needed attention along with strain patterns of the upper arm muscles. Paresthesias of his right thumb and forearm were almost eliminated. He was doing exercises with therabands.

Ten weeks after starting treatment, we began sessions at monthly intervals. Work on the shoulder joint capsule had markedly improved overall joint mobility; and after two more months the inflammation of the bursae was greatly reduced. Localized techniques reduced adhesions of the two ligaments and a nodule in the previously torn region of the trapezoid. I had been working with a blocked, agitated electrical pattern in the ligaments, which was now more calm and balanced. The AC joint capsule was much more normal. At this point Ray was evaluated by the orthopedist, who measured his active shoulder motions at 90 degrees of abduction, 75 degrees of external rotation, and 45 degrees of extension. Each motion was pain-free up to its final 10 degrees. The AC joint still had 15 to 20 percent of instability.

Both mobility and stability continued to improve and eight months after the start of my treatment, Ray had normal range of shoulder motion. The coracoclavicular ligaments had knit together well and the AC joint was at only 5 to 8 percent instability. Strength was much better and he had returned to a regular work pattern. At a follow-up session the following year, the AC joint was even closer to full stability and his shoulder was at full strength and free of pain.

E. Flexor Tendon of Forearm Muscles at Medial Elbow

Felix C. is a 42-year-old acupressure therapist/teacher and fitness trainer. His acupressure work was usually four days a week, but had been limited by an injury to the flexor tendons of his right arm at the elbow. He noticed pain around the medial epicondyle after some months of strenuous rowing on a large lake. He had chiropractic and acupuncture treatment, and not finding much progress, he consulted an orthopedist. The orthopedist identified a torn portion of the tendon and prescribed physiotherapy. After three months of physiotherapy he ordered an MRI, which showed the elbow joint to be relatively normal, but showed a substantial tear in the tendon. Surgical repair was offered as an option.

It was about nine months from the onset of his discomfort when Felix first consulted me. At this point his acupressure work was at half of his normal schedule. There was some pain in proximal portions of his flexor carpi ulnaris, flexor carpi radialis, and pronator teres muscles. He had a normal range of elbow and wrist motion but had pain on passive motions of full elbow and wrist flexion, pronation, supination, and especially in the latter half of wrist extension. There was significant weakness of flexion and extension. At four weekly sessions I worked to reduce swelling of the tendon area and to improve the condition of a zone of the tendon tissue that had a palpable defect of one-half to two-thirds of a centimeter. It was important to employ techniques for reducing excessive tension in the forearm flexor muscles and the biceps and brachialis muscles, because all of these patterns were contributing to undue strain on the injured tendon. Swelling of the tendon area subsided.

At three ensuing bi-weekly sessions I used techniques to improve alignment of the elbow and wrist joints. Felix's upper ribs, thoracic and cervical spine, cranial base and upper abdominal viscera had restrictions that I addressed. His forearm and elbow had a habitual pronation pull, causing a rotational twist that exacerbated irritation of the tendon. I freed restrictions deep to the triceps muscle. There were also important restrictions of the fascia and joint capsule over the coronoid process of the ulna. The tendon fibers were re-aligned and the defect was lessening. Felix increased his acupressure work 25 percent, which was fine as long as he maintained hand and forearm positions that were not too far from neutral position—especially when exerting much pressure.

We switched to three-week intervals and after two more sessions, changed to monthly intervals. Four months after treatment had started, Felix was progressing well with moderate forearm and hand strengthening exercises. The excessive pronation pattern of his elbow and forearm had been normalized. During that time Felix saw the orthopedic surgeon, who was quite pleased with his progress.

Eight months after the start of treatment there were no adhesions in the flexor tendon excepting a slight nodule where the defect had healed. There was no longer pain over the medial epicondyle. Felix was working at 90 percent of his former schedule and doing moderate weight training. He continued to improve and was back to full work capacity when I saw him six months afterward.

F. Achilles Tendon

Kay S. is a 57-year-old owner of a real estate agency who consulted me ten months after a left Achilles tendon (tendo-calcaneus) injury. She noticed pain at the end of a European vacation during which she walked extensively in hilly areas. She was evaluated by an orthopedist and a podiatric surgeon. They both diagnosed a substantial tear of the tendon, and inflammation of its sheath. She received two cortisone injections, physiotherapy and acupuncture. When she first started treatment with me, she found all walking painful and was taking anti-inflammatories three times daily.

I found nodules in and around the tendon. There was a zone on its medial margin with a defect in the tissue and adhesions surrounding this spot. This was the site of most of the tearing which at that level was about 40 percent of the thickness of the tendon. Any dorsiflexion of the ankle was painful and its passive motions limited to 10 degrees. There was considerable weakness in toe raises. At five weekly sessions, Fascial Release techniques were utilized to reduce extensive thickening and adhesions in the tendon sheath. I used induction techniques to feed in the distal end of the tendon toward my contact with my other hand, which was condensing both ends of the gastrocnemius and soleus muscles—in order to release tension in the muscles and tendon simultaneously. This technique affects the muscle spindles and the Golgi tendon organs. Non-force adjustments were used to free the lumbar, sacroiliac, and knee joints.

Kay was now able to do some relaxed swimming. She could walk five blocks with mild pain. At three bi-weekly sessions I worked with restrictions of both feet, especially the left cuboid and fifth metatarsal bones. The tendon fibers were being re-aligned, the sheath was thinning out and the area of defect in the tendon was filling in. Kay took anti-inflammatories only occasionally now.

We started sessions at one-month intervals and four months after the beginning of treatment Kay could walk one mile, with mild pain developing only after the latter half of this activity. She was examined by the podiatric surgeon, who was quite pleased with her progress. The ankle had full dorsiflexion, with pain only in the last 50 degrees. Plantarflexion was now normal in its range.

Seven months after the start of treatment, Kay was swimming and walking regularly. The tendon tissue was much more resilient and the adhesions of the sheath were greatly reduced. She could wear flat shoes comfortably at times when she wasn't doing a lot of walking or prolonged standing. Otherwise, a half-inch heel was adequate for comfort. These improvements had been sustained when I saw Kay one and a half years from the beginning of the sessions.

G. Capsular Ligament of Spinal Facet Joint and Spinal Intertransverse Ligament

Daniel B. is a 38-year-old business executive who is co-owner of a consulting firm. He injured his left lower back fourteen months before consulting me. A windsurfing accident involved a sudden forceful twist to his trunk and a fall. MRI findings and exams by two orthopedic surgeons and a physiotherapist revealed a mild disc bulge at L4-5 and a 5 mm gap of the left zygapophyseal (articular facet) joint of L4-5. The corresponding joint on the right had a 1.5 mm gap. They found instability of his joint and symptoms of a left L5 radiculopathy. Daniel had pain from sitting, standing, bending, and walking. There was some weakness of lower limb muscles, and pain and paresthesia in his left foot. One orthopedist recommended surgery.

Daniel chose to try a conservative care approach and was treated with non-steroidal anti-inflammatories and two epidural steroidal blocks. He had chiropractic care and four months of physiotherapy. Improvement from these approaches was not sustained.

I found limitation of lumbar lateral bending and stiffness of the lower thoracic spine. Counterstrain techniques treated the lower thoracic, lumbar, and sacroiliac joints. Fascial Release was helpful for addressing the paraspinal, gluteal and hip areas. At six weekly sessions I employed BMC techniques of feeding in the capsular ligaments of the left L4-5 articular facet joint and the L4-5 intertransverse ligament (which was "stringy" and twisted). The goal here was to reduce instability of this spinal segment involving laxity of these two ligaments. I also worked to lessen stiffness and adhesions in the left iliolumbar ligament.

Daniel still avoided prolonged sitting when possible and continued exercise instruction from the physiotherapist, gradually adding in some swimming and recumbent stationary bicycling. The weekly sessions were followed by eight bi-weekly sessions during which I continued localized work with the facet capsule and other L4-5 ligaments including the ligamentum flavum. I used manual contact with the vertebrae and leverage from the ribs and pelvis to direct forces into the localized zones of the ligaments. Techniques were also employed to harmonize the Cranial Rhythmic Impulse through the lower spine and lower limbs. After four months of the osteopathic treatment, Daniel's leg and foot symptoms were reduced except after substantial activity. The orthopedist found no muscle weakness. The left facet joint felt more stable with motion testing.

After six months of treatment the intertransverse ligament and the facet joint capsule felt normal to me in terms of their tonus, resiliency, and stability. The left side of the joint was better positioned and more stable. Pain and nerve symptoms were markedly reduced and confined to the low back area. At this point we continued sessions at three-week intervals. The L4-5 ligaments continued to be normal one year from the start of treatment, and his overall functioning was about 85 to 90 percent of his previous level.

H. Annular Ligament of Elbow

Felicia M. is a 45-year-old music teacher/pianist who had right arm and wrist pain resulting from a poorly set fracture of the head of the radius, fifteen years earlier. At a recent examination by an orthopedic surgeon involving X-rays, he diagnosed an enlargement of the radial head along with inferior displacement. He found some arthritic change of the elbow joint. All of Felicia's right elbow movements were stiff and limited. Pronation, supination, and extension were limited to about 20 degrees less than normal, and elbow flexion was restricted by 25 degrees. In the years since the fracture, she had been treated with acupuncture, chiropractic and physiotherapy.

I found a major problem with the annular ligament that holds the radial head in place by wrapping around it and attaching to the ulna. The inferior displacement of the radial head had contributed to the ligament's tearing and its subsequent thickening, adhesions, inelasticity, and disorganized fibrous alignment. Soreness of the ligament was a component of Felicia's elbow pain, which could be provoked by movements in any direction. We commenced weekly sessions at which I addressed the specific tissue condition of the annular ligament along with restrictions of the thoracic outlet, cervical spine, and thoracic spine; all of these were involved in a right rotation of her thorax.

Felicia limited her piano playing to one hour/day at this point and minimized her computer usage, which was also an irritant to the arm. At five weekly sessions I worked with constriction of both collateral ligaments of the elbow and some adhesions in other parts of the joint capsule. The elbow problem seemed to have a significant emotional component that surfaced during the initial sessions. It required some re-adjustment for Felicia to accept the increasing mobility of her arm after fifteen years.

At three bi-weekly sessions I noticed that the four major elbow motions had increased in range to about 10 degrees below normal range. The fascias and muscles of the arm were treated for restrictions along with significant attention to re-alignment of the carpal joints. Felicia started instruction to promote more balanced arm and hand usage in piano playing and computer work. A discordant electrical pattern ("static") of the annular ligament tissue had been normalized, and its tissue was gaining resiliency and pliability. Both attachments of the ligament on the ulna were condensing slightly as I worked to normalize position of the radial head.

After four sessions at monthly intervals (seven months from the start of treatment) Felicia had full and much smoother pain-free elbow motion in all four directions. She played the piano up to two hours a day and could use the computer as needed without pain.

She returned for another session after four months and had a slight decrease in her range of elbow extension and some stiffness of the ligament. This responded well to treatment and her comfort level has been good for one year. The enlarged radial head was now positioned more normally. The progression of this case was somewhat slower and the subsequent results affected by the fairly difficult emotional elements associated with Felicia's elbow problem. At times she would discontinue exercising the arm and some stiffness returned. However, she would return for a "tune-up" session and start exercising, and the elbow was back to normal function.

I. Distal Hamstring (Biceps Femoris) Tendon

This is the case that was reported on the second page of Chapter 1. Julia L. is a dancer and co-chair of a dance department at a university. The case report depicts the obstacles she faced, the therapy process for her injury, and her gradual recovery.

J. Hip Joint Ligaments (Pubofemoral, Iliofemoral)

Mary S. is a 45-year-old dance teacher who was very limited by a right hip injury that had occurred several months before I first saw her. She traced the hip pain and limitation to three sessions of strenuous dance movement when she was quite fatigued and cold. At the time she was recovering from a left knee injury that caused her to put more weight onto her right leg. She had chiropractic treatment and then consulted an orthopedist. X-rays of the area revealed a normal hip joint. He suspected iliopectineal bursitis (in the anterior hip region) prescribed anti-inflammatory medication, and referred her to physiotherapy. She was treated for two months and initially had some improvement, but it wasn't sustained after that. She then had massage and acupuncture treatment. At this point walking for more than five to ten minutes was quite uncomfortable.

At Mary's first session I found marked resistance to adduction and external rotation of her femur. All hip joint movements were stiff and provoked pain toward the end range of movement. On palpation I found zones of the anterior hip capsule ligaments (pubofemoral and the medial part of the iliofemoral) that were stringy, swollen, had disorganized fibers, and contained some nodules. The tearing in these ligaments had left zones with discontinuity of the fibers, which showed significant weakening. The posterior capsular ligaments (ischiofemoral and lateral iliofemoral) were very tight and overly fibrous. I used induction and BMC techniques to realign the fibers, release adhesions, and reduce tissue irritation. At four weekly sessions work was also directed to freeing and balancing the sacroiliac, sacrococcygeal, and lumbar spinal joints, and pubic symphysis. Mary could move more easily and now found gentle stretching more useful

At the following three bi-weekly sessions I continued to use osteopathic visceral manipulation to free restrictions and improve mobility in the right pleura, duodenum, bladder, cecum, and right kidney. This work contributed to releasing tension in the psoas muscle. Excessive tensions in the piriformis, both obturators, quadriceps, and adductor muscles also received attention. The ischiofemoral ligament was more pliable and the damaged portions of the pubofemoral and medial iliofemoral ligaments were knitting together, gaining better tone, and were better organized. At the end of this series Mary could walk a half mile on flat ground fairly comfortably. All hip movements were better in range, with the end ranges of adduction and internal rotation continuing to have some restriction and pain. Mary started Pilates exercise with an expert trainer.

We then met for three sessions at which I continued localized work with the hip ligaments and Fascial Release techniques for the thigh, gluteal, and hip rotator muscles. It was helpful to balance the foot, knee, lumbar, and lower thoracic joints. Five months after the start of treatments Mary could walk one and a quarter miles comfortably and was demonstrating more of the movements for her dance students. All hip movements were normal except for the last five degrees of adduction. At a follow-up session (eight months from the start) she had normal strength of her hip muscles and the tissue quality of the ligaments was healthy. When I spoke with her the following year, Mary said that she had returned to her previous dance workouts and was free of pain.

Chapter 7 contains an overall discussion of the case accounts. The accounts are examples for the next chapter's illustration of the essential processes and tissue changes for a tendon or ligament to heal.

CHAPTER 5

Processes and Tissue Changes in Tendon/Ligament Healing— Related to Manual Therapy

Manual therapy can assist the essential processes and tissue changes that occur as a tendon or ligament heals from serious injury. The case studies provide clear instances that dramatize these events. I will now describe these basic beneficial changes and how they may relate to my usage of appropriate methods. A systematic look at the crucial processes here draws a map of the basic healing mechanism in tendons/ligaments.

The second chapter contains a description of the mechanism and process of chronic tendon/ligament injury. This section will illustrate how that can be reversed in the process of recovery. Examples are drawn from the primary case accounts (Janet C., Robert H.). When a method is mentioned the reader may refer to the technique descriptions in Chapter 3. The assertion that the techniques can assist these favorable changes is based on my experience, and on the writings, research, and teaching of some of the theoreticians referenced earlier—and of the clinicians developing and practicing these methods.

While I am outlining various processes and tissue changes, it is important to note that they are complementary and often interdependent. The first process to mention is the *reduction of the excessive cross-linkage* brought about by intermolecular bonding in problematic collagenous tissue. The clinician aims to restore good tissue metabolism and adequate mobility by reducing the adhesions and fibrosis involving: excessive cross-linkage between tendon or ligament fibers, bundles of fibers, and their interfaces with tendon sheaths and joint capsules. This was essential for Janet's fibrosed, thickened Achilles tendon and its sheath.

Cross-linkage is reduced by the restoration of optimal *inter-fiber mobility* (gliding) which is promoted by the strategy of induction that I use in Fascial Release and other osteopathic techniques (see technique descriptions in Chapter 3). Also, gently condensing the ligament enables the disorganization of the problematic fibrous binding pattern, and allows its subsequent healthy reorganization. I find this application of condensing to be congruent with the alternate feeding in and separating outward of the ends of ligaments/tendons used in Body-Mind Centering; this also increases inter-fiber mobility and normalizes cross-linkage. Another BMC technique that is applicable here is to directly separate the fibers perpendicular to their length. Later I will refer to strategies for minimizing tissue inflammation, raising its metabolic rate, and increasing vascularity; all of these help to reduce the "gluing" of excessive cross-linkage.

The *reduction of excessive muscle tension* and *fascial pulls* that strain the tendon or ligament is another process of change that is an important component of injury healing. Robert's thumb ligament was being stressed by muscular and fascial tensions in his hand and forearm muscles. While all of the techniques described in this chapter effect relaxation, one that is worthy of mention is the Counterstrain approach, which enables muscles to return to normal resting length. This is also assisted by my work with Golgi tendon organs.

Fascial Release technique benefits tense muscles as well as normalizing the pulls through the fascial planes (including the periosteum) that tend to intersect at joints. Visceral Manipulation methods for freeing certain structures in the torso often allow the relaxation of reciprocal tension pulls through the fascias connected to the injury site. It is clear that the restoration of balanced structural alignment promoted by all of these methods is helpful in reducing muscular and fascial tensions and thus also contributes to minimizing localized adhesions.

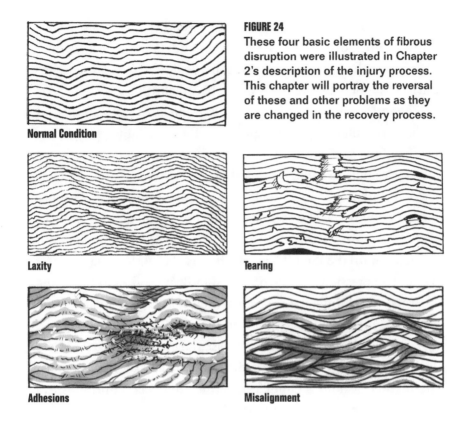

Normal Condition

Laxity

Tearing

Adhesions

Misalignment

FIGURE 24
These four basic elements of fibrous disruption were illustrated in Chapter 2's description of the injury process. This chapter will portray the reversal of these and other problems as they are changed in the recovery process.

The *restoration of normal joint mechanics* to the contiguous joint of a chronically injured tendon/ligament is a vital part of recovery, bringing major benefits for neural, circulatory, and kinesiological functions. Establishing normal mechanics includes the restoration of correct alignment, proper stability, balanced forces in the surrounding ligaments, and normal mobility of the joint. I assisted all these elements for Janet's restricted ankle joint adjacent to the injured tendon by using the methods in the next paragraph.

Counterstrain positionings treat joint dysfunctions through re-establishment of coherent patterns of afferent input. The fulcrums of Zero Balancing, combined with its compressions and tractions, are directly aimed at the normalization of joint function. I find that specific usage of the tissue work of Fascial Release and BMC that corrects restrictions and adhesions of the joint capsule is also beneficial for joint movement. The clinician addresses what Greenman describes as the three findings of somatic dysfunction: asymmetry, restricted motion, and tissue texture abnormality.[87]

The restoration of *adequate blood flow* and *blood/lymph drainage* in the localized injury area is important. This is vital for proper *oxygenation* of the area. Good fluid mechanics are promoted by reduction of excessive muscle and fascial tensions, improvement of nearby joint function, and proper alignment and mobility of the tendon/ligament fibers. I employ specific techniques for improvement of overall and localized circulatory function such as the gentle rhythmic pumping directed toward the fluid flows, which is used in BMC, and the intermittent compression and traction used in BMC and Zero Balancing.

Proper fluid drainage is instrumental for *reducing inflammation,* which is a vital part of the injury healing process. Even though her injury was no longer in the acute phase, Janet's Achilles tendon area remained swollen from inflammation and inadequate fluid drainage. Elimination of fluid accumulations (including sero-fibrinous exudate, see Chapter 2) has many benefits for reducing irritation of the tissues. Reduction of inflammation is also promoted by Counterstrain and all the other techniques I employ to reduce pressure on the tendon/ligament and adjacent areas.

Good circulation also favors the *health and abundance of the ground substance* in the ligament/tendon. This allows an increase in the ratio of its ground substance to the fibers, which is beneficial for tissue mobility and proper metabolism. This production of ground substance is stimulated by movement (after immobilization of an injury) such as intermittent tractions. The favorable condition of adequate fluidity and ductility of the ground substance ("more sol than gel") is enhanced by raising its energy level through techniques that increase its heat, pressure, and level of electromagnetic energy. Some strategies for raising local tissue energy levels are the applications of rhythmic movement and of gentle, direct pressure to the area. Robert's thumb ligament fibers had zones of stiffness and lack of resiliency around the areas of tearing. As the ground substance of the ligament became more abundant and ductile, my palpatory sense of the tissue was that it felt more resilient, bouncy, and "juicy."

Re-establishing the normal parallel arrangement of the tendon/ligament fibers enables efficient functioning and tissue healing. This process is favored by the reduction of excessive cross-linkage of fibers and their bundles, by returning the injured tendon/ligament to its proper length, and by normalizing its electromagnetic condition. The injured structures in the case accounts had generalized disruption of fibrous alignment; there were specific zones where the fibers were noticeably twisted, particularly in proximity to the areas of tearing.

Rearrangement into parallel alignment is aided through encouraging what Bainbridge Cohen calls "hooking" of the fibers, wherein they assume their natural organization in relation to one another. This inherent organization is promoted when I feed in the ends of the ligament toward each other and by the induction used in cranial osteopathy and Fascial Release techniques. It is also encouraged with my usage of very careful manual stretching of the ligament, combined with induction.

This moderate stretching is a form of the passive mobilization that the researcher S.L. Woo believes will promote the *proper remodeling of injured connective tissue* structures such as tendons.[3] Local remodeling is also promoted by restoring overall balanced structural alignment. Parallel fiber arrangement and good vascular function are components of the remodeling mechanism, which incorporates the continuous reorganization process of normal tissue. Tissue remodeling demands the appropriate level of stresses for the tendon, some of which can be provided by manual tractions.

Improvement of neural function is vital for healing of a tendon or ligament. For the localized tendon area this includes 1) releasing pressures on the nerves, 2) reducing excessive proprioceptor activity, 3) lowering "facilitated" (hypersensitive) reflex thresholds to normal levels, and 4) establishing coherent patterns of afferent input.

Fascial Release techniques relieve restrictive pressures along the nerve pathways, thus promoting the neurotrophic flows that provide nourishment to the target tissue. Counterstrain positionings for appropriate spinal joints and for joints near the ligament reduce tissue strains and also reduce excessive proprioceptor activity by means of an approach that is localized and also directed toward the spinal areas. I find these positionings can address what Korr calls segmental dysfunction, which includes the reflex firing patterns involving a spinal segment (cord level, bone and soft tissue) and its circuits to the body's peripheral structures.[16, 88] Segmental stress in Robert's case involved the spine at the thoracic outlet area (particularly C5, C6, C7), which impacted the injured thumb ligament. The injured ligament and its neural receptors are part of this circuit, and the improvement of its receptor activity (afferent input) was enhanced by all of the techniques mentioned in this chapter—some of which decrease the localized nerve irritations caused by the excess fluid pressures and biochemistry of inflammation.

Neural function is also improved through osteopathic cranial and Visceral Manipulation techniques, which reduce reciprocal tension pulls that can pressure the nerve supply to an injured ligament. This aids the ligament by allowing restoration of balanced, undisturbed nerve transmission. Cranial techniques can harmonize the localized structure with the CNS through creating synchrony in the CRI movement patterns that connect them. Cranial techniques also assist in the reduction of overall excessive sympathetic tone, which has several advantages for injury healing.

For some tendons/ligaments that have been immobilized and weakened it is beneficial to increase proprioception as part of their activation. I promote this by using the BMC technique of low-level resistance-pressure, and also through using gentle recoil techniques (rapid release). The recoil consists of the therapist slightly moving the body part into alignment with its force pattern (the pattern of structural pulls in that area), holding it in that position, and quickly releasing his pressure.

As a connective tissue structure such as a tendon or ligament is healing it tends to shorten unless it has beneficial conditions. The problem is often found after incomplete healing, and needs to be reversed by thinning out areas of "gluing," and lengthening the structure to achieve *adequate extensibility and deformability.* This process is favored by reducing adhesions and scar tissue that contain excessive cross-linkage of tendon fibers and their bundles. My palpatory sense is that these zones of adhesed, "glued" fibers feel thick, clumped-together, shortened, and inelastic. This was most pronounced in the thickened, enlarged portions of Janet's tendon and its sheath. In applying the therapeutic strategies about to be mentioned here (and detailed earlier in the techniques section) I use specific localized contact with the zone to soften, separate, and lengthen the adhesed group of fibers, and combine this with techniques to balance and integrate it with the remainder of the tendon and its surrounding tissues.

Adequate extensibility is promoted by reducing low-grade tissue inflammation (that causes fibrosis), encouraging good fluid mechanics, and a high proportion of ground substance in the tendon/ligament. Visco-elastic structures are ideally stretched (lengthened) through gradual loading while they are heated. The heating may be accomplished through manual pressures that raise tissue energy levels (this also occurs in electromagnetic normalization). Tissue heating and loading is also effected when I use Fascial Release and stretching, Zero Balancing tractions, and the BMC techniques of alternative feeding in and elongating the ends of the ligament and separating the fibers perpendicular to their length. The desired end result is a structure with good pliability and optimal length.

An essential component of tissue healing is the *normalization and harmonizing of its electromagnetic activity.* This process involves smooth, regular magnetic pulsation and full, free movement of electrical current in the tendon and its surroundings. Manual pressure on certain acupuncture points in the injury area and in areas adjacent to it seems to promote this mechanism. The smooth flow of electricity and magnetism is facilitated when I optimize the CRI movement through the area of the injured tendon or ligament. It may also be encouraged by the generalized effect of freeing this CRI movement in the cranial area, and then through the body connecting to the injury area. The specific method that I have developed and used for promoting normalization of electromagnetic activity in a tendon or ligament is described in Chapter 3.

Some injured ligaments or tendons (or portions of them) are weak, lax, and atrophied. Their recovery process involves *increasing their tone, substance, and thickness.* I have seen this enable lax structures to regain a more normal length. Minimizing adhesions and scar tissue formation is beneficial due to this tissue's deficiency in elasticity and strength. It is helpful to re-establish proper movement capability of the injured structure both internally and in relation to its surrounding tissues; it has been found that tendon/ligament response to nonexcessive intermittent forces is an increase in thickness and strength.[1] Robert's thumb ligament needed work to correct an overall weakness and laxity and localized zones of thinning and "stringiness" of the fibers. This had resulted from extensive tearing of the ligament.

Manual techniques that I use for increasing tone are the BMC methods of using one's hand on the injured structure to aid the tissue in knitting together, and feeding in the ends of the tendon or ligament toward its center. Some of my focus in the process is on the perpendicular element of the interrelation of the fibers. These techniques can effect weaving together (length-wise and width-wise), thickening, and increased tone. These methods appear to encourage *tissue contractility* (involving the acto-myosin motor, see Chapter 2), which favors a strengthened, more highly toned tendon or ligament. I also utilize Bainbridge Cohen's approach of increasing proprioception to encourage contractility. Through achieving adequate contractibility and tone the ligament can gradually regain its proper length. Counterstrain positionings and other induction-type methods are helpful for the process of stimulating, integrating, and toning a lax ligament.

The above-mentioned techniques have some shared mechanisms for enhancing increased substance and tissue strength: a) activating and balancing the localized tissues (neurologically, etc.), done in a non-stressful manner that is crucial in that it avoids further damage; b) improving their fluid mechanics; and c) beneficially realigning both their internal components (fibers and their bonds) and the relationship to adjacent structures such as neighboring fascias, etc.

The first chapter contains references to the beneficial effects for healing of *raising the metabolic rate of chronically injured connective tissue* (and mentions factors that may promote this). This higher rate is one of the mechanisms mentioned by Studitskii as encouraging the "plastic state," which is important for tissue repair and regeneration.[50] An increased rate of tissue metabolism may be facilitated by heat generated from manual pressure and from movement.

Likely facilitative influences for increased localized metabolism are: 1) enhanced overall energy levels in the body, 2) the increase and normalization of localized electromagnetic activity, 3) adequate, healthy ground substance in the region, and 4) adequate vascular flow resulting in healthy tissue oxygenation, nutritional supply, and waste product removal. Some influences that can enhance overall body energy levels include this increased vascular flow and a more relaxed, deeper respiration. I have noticed that structural improvements resulting from manual therapy directly benefit circulatory and respiratory function and also enable the patient to increase exercise levels, which further promote this energy-enhancing effect. Both Robert and Janet became progressively more active in a comfortable range as they improved. There seemed to be a confluence of enhanced overall energy levels with increased usage, tissue health, and circulatory function of the injury areas. I used Fascial Release and related techniques that free a tendon or ligament from excessive mechanical pressures and improve its circulatory activity, thus benefiting localized tissue metabolism of the injury area.

All of the four factors mentioned in the preceding paragraph (as well as heightened tissue metabolism itself) appear to encourage the *"plastic state"* of the injured structure, which enhances repair and regeneration. This state is described in Chapter 2. The neural function involved with the recovering ligament or tendon is also an important influence in creating a plastic condition.[50]

Healthy, strong nerve currents and neurotrophic supply apparently encourage a plastic condition of the tissue. Research by Becker and others shows that tissue repair capability is boosted by enhanced nerve currents, including the DC flows.[33, 101] My use of acupressure and Zero Balancing techniques that free the movement of acupuncture energy through the tendon area is helpful, as the meridians have been found to conduct DC current[43] (see Chapter 2). Neural function can be enhanced by use of the techniques described in the discussion of its improvement earlier in this section. Heightened nerve activity that may promote the plastic state in the tendon tissue is also stimulated by manual pressures and movement for adjacent areas and contralateral areas, which cause the activation of conditioned reflexes.

This section constructs a map of the processes and tissue changes occurring in tendon/ligament recovery and shows that they are complementary and often interdependent. The final chapter lists these shifts in a further discussion of all the case studies. Recovery progression for the people in the studies involved all of the beneficial changes I have depicted here, facilitated by manual therapy. Interweaving of these functional and structural events portrays essential elements of the healing process.

CHAPTER 6

Self-Help Strategies

Here are some basic strategies of self-help for people with chronic injury of a ligament or tendon. In cases of serious injury this is not a substitute for professional help, although it can be a good adjunct. Some of these methods are not appropriate in the acute stage with the presence of marked inflammation indicated by localized redness, swelling, heat, or a high degree of pain. The strategies are:

- Splinting devices, braces, and supports are often unnecessary in the chronic stage of injury. They can be very useful for the acute stage where restricting motion (e.g. a brace for a recent ankle sprain) is extremely helpful. In chronic cases they can be beneficial for: serving as protection of serious injuries with major fibrous rupture; unavoidable activity that is strenuous and/or repetitive; and preventing undue pressure or strain from stretching or twisting during sleep.

  For chronic injuries be sure that the brace doesn't unduly restrict motion or prevent circulation if you are using it for any length of time. It is best to seek professional advice about getting the proper device. After the acute stage a brace should be used only when necessary, because prolonged immobilization causes problems.

- A note here is that if you suspect that you have a serious injury (with major tearing) of a ligament or tendon, have it assessed by a professional. At the very least this will give you some guidelines for how protective you must be in using that part of your body. An indication of possible serious injury is that the problem area feels unstable and weak.

- Adequate rest is *vital* to recovery. You will have to limit activity for the injury area until it can be tolerated. Injured areas need more time than normal to recuperate after usage.

- Maintain good nutrition, avoiding large amounts of junk food. This is basic and from there one may want to utilize supplements. Substances that appear to have helped in some cases are vitamins, herbs, minerals, homeopathic remedies, and proteolytic enzymes to eliminate the by-products of inflammation. Although I feel some of his supplementation amounts may not be necessary, there is useful information in writings by the nutritional chemist Luke Bucci. One of his more technical books has been referenced in Chapter 2,[99] and for general readers there is *Pain Free* from The Summit Group in Fort Worth, Texas.

- Salves and ointments can be helpful, especially if the injured structure is close to the skin surface. I have seen benefit from certain homeopathic and Chinese medicine preparations. Consult a practitioner to determine if and when their use will be helpful, as this needs to be varied for individual circumstances. Homeopathic salves for injured connective tissue often contain arnica or ruta. Common Chinese medicine preparations are White Flower Oil, Zheng Gu Shui, and Tiger Balm. The more pungent Chinese formulas do not combine well with use of homeopathic remedies.

- When the area around the ligament or tendon is swollen (even in a chronic case) it is helpful to minimize this excess fluid accumulation. When the area is past the acute stage and no longer "hot," frequent *gentle* movement can promote drainage. There are a variety of anti-inflammatory herbs and supplements (and in more acute cases, pharmaceuticals). It is beneficial to avoid pooling of the fluids by elevating the area periodically. Application of cold can be effective particularly after exercise or in alternation with heat (e.g. contrast baths).

• Maintain good circulation in the tendon or ligament, which even in normal conditions does not have much blood supply. When the injury is past the acute stage, good circulation can be promoted by some of the strategies for minimizing swelling (contrast baths, frequent brief periods of gentle movement). Enhancement of overall body circulation through aerobic exercise also helps locally. It can be useful to keep the area warm by covering it with a natural fabric wrap, particularly at night. An example is to use a cut-off sock to fit over the area of an elbow tendon, making sure it is loose enough to permit full circulation.

• Learn to find a baseline for experiencing the area around the ligament or tendon as fully relaxed. Prolonged excessive tension around an injury is very common and is an obstacle to recovery. Relaxation of the area can be enhanced by mild heat (sometimes in alternation with cold), exercise involving the whole body, use of imagery, baths, biofeedback, or meditation. A skilled manual therapy session can deeply relax the area. Once you experience this, you can monitor the area on an ongoing basis with this baseline as a comparison to sense when it is doing well or becoming overly tight. Your memory of the relaxed state is a body experience and recalling it will reduce tension.

• Learn to improve body mechanics for usage of the local area of the tendon or ligament. There are some good self-help guides to ergonomics that are attentive to postural alignment and materials such as furniture and workstation. Reducing strain from poor postural and habitual usage patterns is important. Good occupational usage is essential to recovery from work-related injuries. A few classes from a physical or occupational therapist (e.g. a "back school") or other movement/alignment methods such as Alexander, Body-Mind Centering, or Aston-Patterning could be beneficial. Be sure that the teacher or therapist knows about your injury and has worked with others that are similar— and be conservative with exercise.

• Reduce excessive muscle tension around the ligament or tendon. It is important to be able to stretch the muscles in the surrounding region while being sure to use only a *mild* stretch that pulls directly on the injured structure. In some cases of serious injury, no direct stretch is beneficial while fibers are torn, very weak, or lax. Consultation with a professional experienced in rehabilitation will give you guidelines for how to do regional stretches while avoiding harmful pulls on the injury. Avoid bouncing stretches. Stop and/or avoid stretches where you feel pain or burning located in the localized injury area.

For reducing excessive muscle tension there is an alternative when stretching a muscle would harm an injured ligament/tendon that is in close proximity; you can use self-massage to loosen its tension. It is often advisable to do this before initiating stretches that directly involve the painful area. It will make stretching more effective.

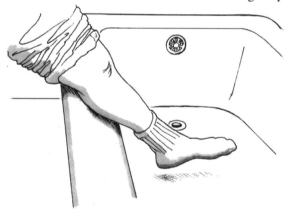

FIGURE 25
Self-massage for calf muscles. Keep lower leg relaxed. Rub and press the leg on the side of the tub or other blunt, stable border. Avoid direct pressure on the injury area or back of knee joint.

Use the hand or a wooden or other mechanical massage device. For the calf muscles you can gently press and rub the fleshy part of the lower leg on the blunt edge of a bathtub, while you keep the leg relaxed and avoid rapid movement. Similar strategies can be improvised for forearm muscles using rounded or padded (with a folded towel) corners of a stable object such as a countertop. Be careful not to directly pressure or put much pull on the injury.

When muscles have habitual zones of congestion you may do well to have them worked out by manual therapy. Skilled massage, Fascial Release, Myofascial therapy and other methods can assist in freeing the tension in these hot spots. A guiding principle here is that the closer the therapist is working to your injured ligament or tendon, the more skill, experience, and respect for damaged tissue is demanded. Manual techniques that are fine for general muscle tension may be harmful when applied to the injury zone.

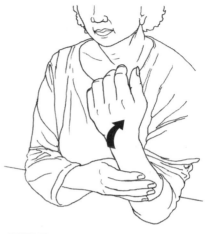

FIGURE 26
Passive stretch for muscles and connective tissue at rear of upper arm and back of elbow. Allow left forearm to remain at rest while you lift it evenly and slowly. Stretches such as this are most beneficial when applied with an element of rotation (arrow), which avoids your compressing the forearm directly into the elbow joint.

- Passive stretch for a muscle, ligament, or tendon is done with aid of an outside force. An example is using your hand to bend (flex) the opposite elbow by pulling the resting forearm up toward the shoulder (see Figure 26). Controlled passive motion stimulates tensile strength of the ligament by helping to increase its collagen content; for this purpose the motion can be passive stretching or motion in other directions. If you are advised that the injured structure will tolerate mild direct stretch to restore its flexibility, gentle passive stretch can be less stressful than active motion. During a stretch, when you have passed the range where the muscle is still elongating, you are then specifically stretching the tendon or ligament. Be very careful. The feeling of stretching a healthy ligament or tendon is of gradual resistance with a firm but yielding quality.

• Resistance exercise to strengthen the region of the injury can be beneficial to restore stability. It can help restore normal tone to the ligament fibers and increase muscular support from the surrounding area. This is only appropriate after the acute stage. For some injuries a significant level of direct resistance pressure is well tolerated only after a substantial portion of the healing process is established. Start with a light weight and be patient. Resistance exercise directly involving the injury area demands caution and you should get advice from an expert in rehabilitation on when and how to do it properly. In my experience, even some health professionals are too aggressive in recommending this type of exercise. It is all too easy to overdo and reverse your progress.

Therabands and light weights are common aids for strength training. Resistance for muscle groups not directly involving the injury area can of course be started earlier. For people with low muscle tone, the stability provided by strengthening is quite important. If the tendon or ligament feels sore during exercise it isn't right for you. If the habitual soreness of the area is increased that night or the next morning, you may have done too much. It is definitely too much if there is sharp pain or if pain remains in the injured structure twenty-four hours after resistance or any other exercise.

• Cardiovascular exercise promotes tendon/ligament healing by improving overall circulation, breathing, and metabolism. It also helps these functions locally. As long as the movement doesn't strain the injury area, some form of this activity (e.g. walking, cycling, swimming) will aid your recovery. If your work or lifestyle is sedentary, frequent brief periods of gentle movement are helpful.

- Proprioceptive sensations provide information about the position, movement, and equilibrium of the body and its various regions. This vital communication function of the nervous system is disrupted in the injury process. Re-establishing good proprioception in the area of injury (which will then relay appropriate signals to the brain) will be important for your recovery. An excellent strategy for leg problems (knee, ankle, etc.) is to stand on an unstable surface such as a balance board or some thick foam. Toe raises supported on both feet or one foot serve a similar purpose. Feldenkrais exercise or resistance exercises with free weights or therabands are helpful for restoring healthy proprioception.

Coming back from serious injury is in some ways a journey, and you can learn about the ligament or tendon and capacities you have for moving toward full recovery.

CHAPTER 7

Conclusions

"Osteopathy is the art of provoking self-correction
on the part of the organism."[67]

The course of this book illustrates a new approach to tendon/ligament healing. The therapy model I've developed is shown in action for treatment in the injury cases. The reader also sees an unusual view of the nature of these connective tissue structures.

This chapter highlights the two peoples' cases reported in depth in Chapter 4. I will relate them to tendon/ligament healing capacity, essential changes in their recovery process, and the role of manual therapy. Other major features of the book to be viewed here in light of the cases include basic principles of structural health care, and the research study of effectiveness (outlined earlier). This chapter also contains further thoughts on clinical efficacy, which involves important capabilities of a therapist for success with serious injuries. Part of the concluding summary is a look at directions in this health care area.

Discussion of the Cases, Overview

The accounts trace healing from chronic injuries of tendons and ligaments, with help from the structural/osteopathic manual therapy that I provided. The data used are my clinical notes, the patients' reports of their condition, the reports of other clinicians, and reports of MRI findings. Discussion here contains examples from the two in-depth case accounts in Chapter 4, which contain all the essential features of the topic. The ten capsule case reports at the end of that chapter have a similar pattern to the detailed cases, and substantiate their findings. In some general instances I will refer to "all twelve" or "all" cases.

Each person's account traces progress of several variables during the course of treatment. These variables are: 1) level of comfort/pain, 2) range of motion of the joint(s) adjacent to the injury, 3) capacity for function, and 4) clinical findings such as tissue quality of the tendon/ligament (resiliency, tone, stability, etc.). In each of the twelve cases the various data sources showing progression of the different variables all indicate the subjects' consistent, gradual normalization and return to healthy condition.

The two people (Janet and Robert) in the basic cases had positive and negative indicators in their potential for recovery. Their age (both in their forties) was in the middle range for healing capacity, relative to a much younger or older person. Some other major indicators were average or above, and these include: having good overall health, adequate nutrition, a relatively stable emotional pattern, and willingness to cooperative with a treatment program. However, both injuries were quite serious—with significant tearing of fibers, other tissue damage, loss of function, very little responsiveness to other forms of treatment, chronic duration, and recommendation for surgery in both cases. Their prognosis for complete recovery with surgery was uncertain. Injuries of this nature are not unusual; there is a high incidence of occupational and other disability from them.

The subjects in the cases in response to manual therapy, appeared to demonstrate properties of tendons/ligaments which are favorable for recovery from chronic injury (see Chapter 2). These properties are: 1) significant capacity for tissue contractility, 2) a continual remodeling (self-renovation) process of connective tissue that is more extensive than in the conventional model, 3) substantial innervation of tendons/ligaments and its contribution to their influential postural and movement role (this role was improved in both cases), and 4) a capacity for healing, also more pronounced than in the conventional medical model. There seemed to be an improvement in their electrical and magnetic activity; this may exemplify the property of being responsive to electromagnetism.

While both people in the in-depth accounts exhibited all the primary aspects of serious injury and the recovery process, the two have a different emphasis. Recovery for Janet's Achilles tendon is notable for reduction of very substantial thickening, adhesion, and excessive cross-linkage of its fibers. The surrounding fascias including the tendon sheath were major structural factors here with their abnormal "gluing" to the tendon. A large nodule in the tendon was gradually normalized through the manual treatment. Janet had a very painful injury and recovery involved a decrease of hyper-reactivity of the tendon tissue. A key to restoring her range of motion was reducing fibrosity and cross-linkage, while in Robert's case the main limitation was from pain and caution about weakness.

In Robert's recovery, his chronically weak, lax, overstretched ligament regained good tone, length, substance, and strength. This was the most striking evidence of change. I worked to normalize thinness and "stringiness" of the fibers. The thumb ligament went through a process of restoration in regions that had very substantial tearing and wasting of fibers. Overall, his was a more fragile structure than Janet's tendon, although this had also incurred significant rupture of fibers and neural disruption. A particular challenge for Robert's progress was demanding occupational usage for his injured hand.

Similar features of the two cases were that the injured tendon and ligament needed correction for major misalignment of normal parallel fiber arrangement. In both Janet's and Robert's situation the structure had nodules, thickened areas and swelling. I utilized methods in each case to improve stiffness and lack of resiliency of the tissue. As they progressed, structural improvement enabled increased exercise levels leading to better circulatory and respiratory function. A resulting increase of overall bodily energy levels correlated with greater usage, better metabolism, and tissue health of the injury zone. Rest, usage with balanced alignment, and appropriate exercise were important to each person's recovery. The subjects were generally cooperative in these areas.

A basic feature of my therapy approach for all twelve people (seen in detail in the two primary accounts) were techniques to specifically and directly alter the structure of the tendon/ligament, including its microstructure (e.g. fiber re-alignment). Another basic is balancing the joints around it which were the ankle, knee and foot joints for the Achilles tendon, and the thumb, hand and wrist joints for the thumb ligament. Also, strategies to address the cranial, spinal and visceral structures and their associated rhythms (e.g. CRI) are part of a whole body approach; one goal of this is to remove connecting pulls on the injury area.

All the subjects noticed major improvement (to normal levels) of their function, comfort, and range of motion. They reported that this healthy condition was still present nine months to three years after completion of treatment. Other clinicians who had treated them also noticed these improvements, as well as healthier tissue quality of the tendon/ligament, reduced inflammation, and better function of the contiguous joint.

Processes and tissue changes that occur as a tendon or ligament heals from chronic injury (and their relation to certain manual therapy methods) are described in Chapter 5. Those that I *directly observed* for the injured tendon/ligament in all case progressions were:

- reduction of excessive cross-linkage and adhesion of its fibers, bundles of fibers, and surrounding structures
- reduction of excessive muscular and fascial pulls on it
- restoration of normal mechanics to its contiguous joint(s)
- improved vascular flow through the area
- reduced inflammation

- restoration of its normal parallel fiber arrangement
- improved, normalized neural function (e.g. localized decrease of hyper-reactivity)
- restoration of adequate length, deformability (pliability) and extensibility
- proper modeling and remodeling of its tissues
- decreased laxity—increased strength, tone, resiliency.

The following processes and tissue changes for the healing tendon/ligament in the cases were inferred and/or directly observed to a somewhat lesser degree than those listed above:

- a more fluid ground substance
- improved, normalized neural function (e.g. healthier feedback loops and neurotrophic activity)
- improved tissue metabolism and oxygenation
- appearance of a "plastic state" for tissue regeneration
- better lymphatic drainage
- normalization of electromagnetic activity.

A basic bodily healing response was described in Chapter 2, a reaction to injury that may enhance the repair process of any part of the body. Recovery for the people in the case studies appeared to include all the elements of this response. Of the "processes and tissue changes" listed above, those involving tissue re-modeling, neural responses, electromagnetic activity, the "plastic state," tissue metabolism, and vascular/lymphatic function are features of the basic bodily healing mechanism which applied to connective tissue repair for the subjects. I have reported these changes in most detail for the two primary cases.

Treatment of each person's injury includes all of the osteopathic and other non-force structural methods of my therapy model for tendons and ligaments. These were described in Chapter 3. The essential principles of these techniques listed below are all seen in the treatment picture. Another common feature is a focus on interrelation of the nervous system with the musculoskeletal system. This is particularly advantageous for treatment of tendons and ligaments, which have extensive neural involvement.

While there may be other effective therapeutic strategies for healing in similar situations it certainly appears that an in-depth, comprehensive manual therapy approach would be important for good results with serious, chronic injuries. All the people had previously received other forms of manual therapy and other conservative care without success.

There are some common essential principles of the techniques in this model which are demonstrated in the case accounts.

- Normalizing force patterns and reciprocal tension pulls in the body—combined with precise attention to localized centers of dysfunction and stress.

- Harmonizing the peripheral structures (i.e. tendon/ligament) with the center of the body and CNS (through the vertebral column and cranium).

- Re-establishing movement that is balanced and unobstructed is basic to (structural) health.

- There are intrinsic movement and force patterns in the body (i.e. CRI and optimal fluid circulation). Facilitating these patterns to operate freely is beneficial.

- Encouraging self-correction in the body. This is founded on a belief in the intelligence of the body, down to its minute components. When given the opportunity it is a self-correcting organism.

- Usage of small, well-targeted changes (e.g. at the foci of physiological patterns) can have a major impact when the clinician comprehends the overall structure and dynamic.

- Combination of direct and indirect approach, with extensive usage of indirect techniques, in which the therapist follows the body's structural and movement inclination.

It is important to acknowledge the potential positive influence of nutritional strategies (including dietary and herbal supplements), stress reduction, and skilled movement therapy to promote connective tissue healing. These can be quite effective and can be useful in combination with manual therapy.

In general my approach is best-suited to injured areas which are mostly accessible to direct touch, such as those in the case studies. While the progress is slower, there have also been good results with more obscured, deeply situated structures (e.g. deeply placed spinal ligaments, see Daniel B.'s case G). It is easiest when the tissues are directly palpable, however many of the techniques (Counterstrain, BMC, Fascial Release) are also quite useful for tendons/ligaments with limited direct access.

Timing of the sessions can be important. For this style of therapy, which aims to promote significant structural change at each session, it is beneficial to allow at least a one-week interval. Overly frequent sessions may irritate vulnerable structures and can prevent adequate integration of previous changes.

A positive factor influencing recovery is a good rapport between the clinician and client. This includes confidence, sense of common direction, and timely use of humor. A good (or sometimes not-so-good) joke can be quite helpful.

A summary of the research design aspect of the book (see Chapter 4) follows for readers interested in this area. The case study design is meant to measure the efficacy of my approach. There appears to be a strong correlation between usage of the manual techniques and beneficial change for all twelve subjects.

In regard to the capacity for use of this model of manual therapy to effect injury healing for tendons/ligaments, the research design is not intended to provide proof through statistical generalization (randomized sampling). However, the case reports in context do demonstrate validation of therapeutic efficacy through analytical generalization, which relates a particular set of results (recovery from injury during therapy) to a broader model (the therapeutic model I use). Along with this deductive approach the research data establishes validation through the inductive analysis approach—which starts with specific empirical observation (recovery from injury during therapy) and builds toward a general pattern.

Multiple sources of evidence have been utilized to trace a set of variables over time, leading to the same conclusion (triangulation). This is illustrated in the progression charts at the end of both primary cases. Context is established by relating my work to the most widely used approach (standard medical) and discussing clinical theory, positive/negative indicators for success in the cases, and ways to minimize the researcher's bias. A section in Chapter 3 describes the training and experience I've had for developing technical and perceptual skills utilized to apply the clinical techniques. In sum, this supports predictive value for the case study research; usage of this therapeutic model in similar cases is likely to provide considerable assistance in recovery.

Further Thoughts on Clinical Efficacy

What are the crucial elements of my therapy approach that enable positive results in cases of serious and chronic injury? Although the combination of techniques that I use is unusual, there are other practitioners who utilize some or most of them and yet may not be effecting this kind of result in general. The case studies involve recovery for tendons and ligaments with substantial tearing and other damage, and loss of function—which had previously been unresponsive to treatment.

One element that is clearly vital for success is thorough training in the manual techniques, including instruction from expert teachers. I have combined instruction with independent study, clinical practice, and my own teaching to further knowledge of the methods. There is not an effective alternative to solid technical training along with experience.

What else enables me to effectively use these techniques for a good outcome in difficult cases? We should emphasize the importance of the therapist as instrument, not just a mechanical tool but with accurately responsive action and perception. The skill of "listening" consists of the practitioner allowing his hand to be drawn to the center of dysfunctional structural patterns in the body as a whole, and in localized regions. Application of this valuable diagnostic method is greatly enhanced by awareness training (there is some description of this in the reference to "sensing" in the personal background section). The awareness practice is fundamental to my clinical work. It aids the capacity to synchronize and center my focus through a state of attentive, balanced relaxation of my own body while working.

Awareness is a crucial factor in consistent clinical application of an alert, observational focus that I use in diagnosis and in carrying out the treatment techniques. This focus involves a type of listening that is an active receptivity utilized in monitoring the patient's body. It enables effective adjustment in the course of applying a technique and fine-tuning of the treatment while in progress. During the treatment session I may perceive that a strain pattern (unbalanced pull) is coming from within the bone in the injury area. Or the force line of the strain pattern is found to be originating in one of the various specific tissue levels (such as periosteum, cartilage, tendon sheath, etc.) that wasn't apparent at first, but is important to address. Attentiveness allows precision in tracing body patterns to locate focal centers of structural dysfunction; and precision in promoting their beneficial change which has important overall benefit including recovery from injury.

An alert observational focus enables accuracy in both diagnostic and treatment procedures. An important component of diagnosis is attunement to the basic body rhythms of the patient, which I also use in applying the techniques. The attunement is made possible by the capacity of listening that enables the practitioner to establish contact with the body while disturbing its function as little as possible. An example of the value of ability to utilize a finely tuned, precise, therapeutic approach is that a large amount of the benefit of Counterstrain positioning occurs in locating the final half to quarter inch of an exactly correct position of release for a joint. This is also primary for structurally detailed work with the microstructure of connective tissue.

I do not intend this discussion of important capabilities to sound esoteric or overly mysterious. The capacity to be attentive on an ongoing basis (including awareness of subtle change of structure) is vital to what I do. Emphasis here is on development of the operator as instrument, not just an interchangeable mechanical part but with a clear, actively perceptive focus.

This perception and action is more clinically accurate and useful when combined with a thorough knowledge of anatomy and kinesiology. An ongoing interest in anatomy has led to continuing study that has significant application in practice. Anatomical study that includes an experiential dimension (capacity to identify and sense the structures within one's own body) seems to further enhance therapeutic efficacy. Familiarity with the body through movement derived from participation in sports, dance, and physical work (this includes the work of my clinical practice) has been very instructive and helpful in dealing with the area of a patient's physical functioning.

Another element involving personal experience that has been very useful in treating complicated cases is my own recovery from the serious, chronic tendon injury described in the "background" section of Chapter 3. The experience of finding a way to recover has deep-ened knowledge, insight, and confidence. It has strengthened a long-term belief in the plasticity of the body. This attitude that the tissue is dynamic and responsive is a motivation to be persistent in finding strategies to improve a condition even when it is ingrained. Patience and persistence in clinical problem-solving is central.

Practicing since 1973 has given me extensive opportunity to thor-oughly learn and experiment with different therapies and to determine if and when each is appropriate. Longevity of experience has afforded the advantage of seeing many different clinical situations and responses to treatment, including the emotional aspect; this is another key ele-ment of the capacity to achieve good results in difficult injury cases.

It is not my intention that practitioners will incorporate all of this therapy model, but that they may want to explore and utilize some of its elements.

Concluding Summary. Directions in This Health Field

The approach I've developed is a therapy model for tendon/ligament healing. The model is a synthesis of various manual techniques with a particular way of applying them involving capacities of the thera-pist (featured in the preceding section on "efficacy").

A major goal of this book is to demonstrate how subtle and com-plex structural therapy can be done in a systematic, anatomically focused way. There is often a belief that subtle work is completely intuitive and without a technical, anatomical basis. I have aimed to illustrate inte-gration of strong technical/anatomical expertise with perceptual capacity involving attentive focus, for effective clinical work.

This integration is a crucial part of my direction in this field up to the present. Readers have seen that the direction I've taken also includes creative strategy for tissue and microstructure treatment of tendons and ligaments, as well as methods to incorporate their newly found physiological properties into the therapy approach. The properties involve neural response, cellular change, electromagnetism, tissue remodeling, and contractility.

A vital future direction in this health care field is further development combining technical and perceptual skills. I am also presently exploring manual therapy strategies for cartilage injury, which is another challenging area for tissue healing. An important continuing focus is further development of manual methods involving electricity and magnetism.

My feeling is that research on various therapeutic uses of electromagnetism for connective tissue should be of great benefit, as well as other areas of research on regeneration of tendons/ligaments. Exploring the role of satellite cells in this regeneration is very intriguing. Increased integration of manual therapy with standard medicine in the health care system is also an important future direction.

The first chapter raises a variety of possibilities. My goal has been that the book's information on the topics provides a firm grounding for seeing these potentials as realistic and viable:

- Healing capacity of tendons and ligaments that is greater than seen in the standard medical model.
- Essential principles of structural health care with the body as a dynamic, responsive organism.
- Effective role of manual therapy in a new approach to chronic injury.

The book's focus is the solid basis for a sense of possibility that in serious, chronic tendon and ligament injury there are avenues for a vital and natural function that is healing.

List of Illustrations and Photographs

Works Cited

1. Norkin, C. and Levangie, P., *Joint Structure and Function* (F. A. Davis, Philadelphia, 1992).

2. Ganong, W., *Medical Physiology* (Appleton and Lange, Norwalk, Conn., 1992).

3. Woo, S. L.-Y, "Biomechanics of Tendons and Ligaments," *Frontiers in Biomechanics*, Woo, S. L., Schmid-Schonbein, G. W., Zweifach, B. W., eds. (Springer-Verlag, New York, 1986).

4. Kessler, R. and Hertling, D., "Assessment of Musculoskeletal Disorders," *Management of Musculoskeletal Disorders*, Kessler, R. and Hertling, D., eds. (Lippincott, Philadelphia, 1990).

5. Juhan, D., *Job's Body* (Station Hill Press, Barrytown, New York, 1987).

6. Cailliet, R., *Soft Tissue Pain and Disability* (F. A. Davis, Philadelphia, 1996).

7. Frankel, V. and Nordin, M., *Basic Biomechanics of the Skeletal System* (Lea and Febiger, Philadelphia, 1980).

8. Keene, J. S., "Ligament and Muscle-Tendon-Unit Injuries," *Orthopedic and Sports Physical Therapy*, Gould, J. and Davies, G., eds. (Mosby, St. Louis, 1985).

9. Adams, L. M., "The Anatomy of Joints Related to Function," *Mechanics of Human Joints*, Radin, E. L. and Wright, V., eds. (Dekker, New York, 1990).

10. Viidik, A., "Normal Healing of Tendons and Ligaments," *Biomechanics of Diarthrodial Joints*, Mow, V., Ratcliffe, A., Salvio, L., eds (Springer-Verlag, New York, 1990).

11. Seedhom, B., "Ligament Reconstruction: Anterior Cruciate Ligament," *Mechanics of Human Joints*, Radin, E. L. and Wright, V., eds. (Dekker, New York, 1990).

12. Kirkaldy-Willis, W., *Managing Low Back Pain* (Churchill Livingstone, New York, 1990).

13. Paris, S. V., *The Spine*, Course Notes (Atlanta, 1982).

14. Subotnick, S. and Sisney, P., "Treatment of Achilles Tendinopathy in the Athlete," *J. Am. Podiatriac Medical Association.*, 76: 10, 552–556 (1987).

15. Garrick, J. and Radetsky, P., *Peak Fitness* (Crown, New York, 1986).

16. Korr, I. M., *Collected Papers of I. M. Korr* (Amer. Acad. of Osteopathy, Colorado Springs, 1979).

17. Rowinski, M. J., "Afferent Neurobiology of the Joint," *Orthopedic and Sports Physical Therapy*, Gould, J. and Davies, G., eds. (Mosby, St. Louis, 1985).

18. Lehmkuhl, L. D. and Smith, L. K., *Brunnstrom's Clinical Kinesiology* (F.A. Davis, Philadelphia, 1983).

19. Wyke, B. D., "Articular Neurology and Manipulative Therapy," *Aspects of Manipulative Therapy*, Idczak, I. M., ed. (Lincoln Institute of Health Sciences, Victoria, Australia, 1980).

20. Johansson, H. and Sjolander, P., "Neurophysiology of Joints," *Mechanics of Human Joints* Radin E. L. and Wright, V., eds. (Dekker, New York, 1990).

21. Basmajian, J. V. and DeLuca, C., *Muscles Alive* (Williams and Wilkins, Baltimore, 1985).

22. Radin, E. L., "Mechanically-Induced Periarticular and Neuromuscular Problems," *Mechanics of Human Joints*, Radin, E. L. and Wright, V., eds. (Dekker, New York, 1990).

23. Bowling, R. and Rockar, P., "The Elbow Complex," *Orthopedic and Sports Physical Therapy*, Gould, J. and Davies, G., eds. (Mosby, St. Louis, 1985).

24. LeVeau, B. F., "Basic Biomechanics in Sports and Orthopedic Physical Therapy," *Orthopedic and Sports Physical Therapy*, Gould, J. and Davies, G., eds.(Mosby, St. Louis, 1985).

25. Kessler, R., "Friction Massage," *Management of Common Musculoskeletal Disorders*, Kessler, R. and Hertling, D. eds. (Lippincott, Philadelphia, 1990).

26. Viidik, A. and Gottrup, F., "Mechanics of Healing Soft Tissue Wounds," *Frontiers in Biomechanics*, Woo, S. L., Schmid-Schonbein, G. W., Zweifach, B. W., eds. (Springer-Verlag, New York, 1986).

27. Simkin, P. A., "Biology of Joints," *Mechanics of Human Joints*, Radin, E. L. and Wright, V., eds. (Dekker, New York, 1990).

28. Jones, L. H., *Jones Strain-Counterstrain* (Jones Strain-Counterstrain Inc., Boise, Id. 1995).

29. Hertling, D. and Kessler, R., "The Wrist and Hand Complex," *Management of Common Musculoskeletal Disorders*, Kessler, R. and Hertling, D., eds., (Lippincott, Philadelphia, 1990).

30. Rolf, I. P., *Rolfing: The Integration of Human Structures* (Harper and Row, 1977).

31. Korr, I. M., "Proprioceptors and Somatic Dysfunction," *J. Am. Osteop. Association*, 74: 638–650 (1975).

32. Kessler, R., "Arthrology," *Management of Common Musculoskeletal Disorders*, Kessler, R. and Hertling, D., eds., (Lippincott, Philadelphia, 1990).

33. Becker, R. L. and Selden, G., *The Body Electric* (Dekker, New York, 1990).

34. Becker, R. L., *Cross Currents* (Putnam, New York, 1983).

35. Becker, R. L., "Electromagnetism and Life," *Modern Bioelectricity*, Marino, A.A., ed. (Dekker, New York, 1988).

36. Marino, A., ed., *Modern Bioelectricity* (Dekker, New York, 1988).

37. Williamson, S. J., ed., *Biomagnetism: An Interdisciplinary Approach* (Plenum, New York, 1983).

38. Sisken, B., "Effects of Electromagnetic Fields on Nerve Regeneration," *Modern Bioelectricity*, Marino, A. A., ed. (Dekker, New York, 1988).

39. Smith, S., "Limb Regeneration," *Modern Bioelectricity*, Marino, A. A., ed. (Dekker, New York, 1990).

40. Gerber, R., *Vibrational Medicine* (Bear and Co., Santa Fe, 1988).

41. Lackie, J. M., ed., *Cell Movement and Cell Behavior* (Allen and Unwin, London, 1986).

42. Hunt, V., *Infinite Mind: The Science of Human Vibrations* (Malibu, Malibu, Ca., 1995).

43. Reichmanis, M., "Electro-acupuncture," *Modern Bioelectricity*, Marino, A. A., ed. (Dekker, New York, 1988).

44. Abercrombie, M. and Dunn, G. A., "Locomotion and Contraction in Nonmuscle Cells," *Contractile Systems in Nonmuscle Tissues*, Perry S. V. and Margreth, A., eds. (Elsevier, Amsterdam, 1976).

45. Elzinga, M. and Lu, R., "Comparative Amino Acid Sequence Studies on Actin," *Contractile Systems in Nonmuscle Tissues*, Perry, S.V. and Margreth, A., eds. (Elsevier, Amsterdam, 1976).

46. Pollard, T. and Fujiwara, K., eds., "Participation of Contractile Proteins in Cytoplasmic Stractive and Cell Division," Perry, S. V. and Margreth, A., eds., *Contractile Systems in Nonmuscle Tissues* (Elsevier, Amsterdam, 1976).

47. Weber, K., "Biochemical Anatomy of Microfilaments of Cells in Tissue Culture," *Contractile Systems in Nonmuscle Tissues* (Elsevier, Amsterdam, 1976).

48. Strohman, R., Yamada, S., Buffinger, N., "Fibroblast Growth Factor Plays a Role in Regulating Muscle Hypertrophy," *Medicine and Science in Sports and Exercise*, Am. Coll. of Sports Medicine S: 173–80 (1989).

49. Strohman, R., Personal Communication (1995).

50. Studitskii, A. N., *Transplantation of Muscles in Animals* (Oxonian, New Delhi, 1988).

51. Schiaffino, S., Bormioli, S., Aloisi, M., "Fiber Branching and Formation of New Fibers During Compensatory Muscle Hypertrophy," *Muscle Regeneration*, Mauro, A., ed. (Raven, New York, 1979).

52. Carlson, B. M., "Muscle Regeneration and Aging,"*Monographs in Developmental Biology*, 23: 189–95 (1992).

53. Moore, M. A., "Stem Cell Concepts," *Muscle Regeneration*, Mauro, A., ed. (Raven, New York, 1979).

54. Butler, D., *Mobilization of the Nervous System* (Churchill Livingstone, Melbourne, 1991).

55. Cohen, B. B., Manuals for Courses in Body-Mind Centering (School for Body-Mind Centering, Amherst, Mass., 1977–1987).

56. Cohen, B. B., Personal Communications (1993–96).

57. Cohen, B. B., *Sensing, Feeling and Action* (Contact Editions, Northampton, Mass, 1993).

58. Kessler, R. and Hertling, D., eds., *Management of Common Musculoskeletal Disorders* (Lippincott, Philadelphia, 1990).

59. Barak, T., Rosen, E., Sofer, R., "Mobility: Passive Orthopedic Manual Therapy," *Orthopedic and Sports Therapy*, Gould J. and Davies, G., eds. (Mosby, St. Louis, 1985).

60. Dyson, M., "Stimulation of Tissue Repair by Ultrasound, *Physiotherapy*, 64: 105–8 (1978).

61. Forster, A., Palastanga, N., *Clayton's Electrotherapy*, (Bailliere Tindall, London, 1982).

62. Palastanga, N., "Transverse Friction Massage," *Modern Manual Therapy of the Vertebral Column*, Grieve, G. P., ed. (Churchill Livingstone, Edinburgh, 1986).

63. Radin E. L., "Osteoarthrosis," *Mechanics of Human Joints*, Radin, E. L. and Wright, V. eds. (Dekker, New York, 1990).

64. Jones, L. H., Seminars, Strain-Counterstrain (1987, 1991).

65. College of Osteopathic Medicine of the Pacific, Cranial Course Manual (1985).

66. Becker, Rol., "Diagnostic Touch I and II," *Yearbooks, Academy of Applied Osteopathy*, (1963 and 1964).

67. Barral, J. P., *Visceral Manipulation* (Eastland, Seattle, 1987).

68. McPartland, J. M. and Mein, E. A., "Entrainment and the Cranial Rhythmic Impulse," *J. Alternative Therapies in Health and Medicine* 1: 40–46 (1997).

69. Smith, F. F., Seminars, Zero Balancing (1981–3).

70. Lippincott, H. and R., *Manual of Cranial Technique* (Edwards Brothers, Ann Arbor, 1943).

71. Magoun, H. I., *Osteopathy in the Cranial Field* (Journal Printing, Kirksville, Mo., 1966).

72. Barral, J. P., *Visceral Manipulation II* (Eastland, Seattle, 1987).

73. Sutherland, W. G., *The Cranial Bowl* (Free Press, Mankato, Minn., 1939).

74. Barral, J. P., *Manual Thermal Diagnosis* (Eastland, Seattle, 1996).

75. Jones, L. H., "Spontaneous Release by Positioning," DO 4: 109–16 (1964).

76. Frymann, V. M., "A Study of the Rhythmic Motions of the Living Cranium," *J. Am. Osteopath Assoc.* 70: 928–45 (1971).

77. Gehin, A., *Atlas of Manipulative Techniques for the Cranium and Face* (Eastland Press, Seattle, 1985).

78. Cohen, B. B., Seminar, Fluid System, School for Body-Mind Centering (1995).

79. Barral, J. P., *The Thorax* (Eastland, Seattle, 1989).

80. Barral, J. P., *Urogenital Manipulation* (Eastland, Seattle, 1993).

81. Barral, J. P., Seminars, Visceral Manipulation (1986–93).

82. Smith, F. F., *Inner Bridges* (Humanics, Atlanta, 1990).

83. Austin M., *Acupuncture Therapy* (ASI Publishers, New York, 1972).

84. College of Osteopathic Medicine of the Pacific, Manual of Fascial Release Techniques (1984).

85. Becker, F., "The Meaning of Fascia and Fascial Continuity," *Osteopathic Annals* 35–47 (June, 1975).

86. Walther, D. S., *Applied Kinesiology Synopsis* (Systems D. C., Pueblo, Co., 1988).

87. Greenman, P. E., In *Neurobiologic Mechanisms in Manipulative Therapy*, Korr, I. M., ed. (Plenum, New York, 1979).

88. Patterson, M. M., In *Neurobiologic Mechanisms in Manipulative Therapy*, Korr, I. M., ed. (Plenum, New York, 1979).

89. Yin, R. K., *Case Study Research* (Sage, Thousand Oaks, Ca., 1994).

90. Polkinghorne, D. E., *Phenomenological Research Methods* (Plenum, New York, 1987).

91. Nachmias, D. and Nachmias, C., *Research Methods* (Plenum, New York, 1987).

92. Patton, M. Q., *Qualitative Evaluation and Research Methods* (Sage, Newbury Park, Ca., 1990).

93. Miles, M. B. and Huberman, A. M., *Qualitative Data Analysis* (Sage, Newbury Park, Ca., 1994).

94. Merriam, S. B., *Case Study Research in Education* (Sage, Newbury Park, Ca., 1988).

95. Hoppenfeld, S., *Physical Examination of the Spine and Extremities* (Appleton-Century, Norwalk, Conn., 1976).

96. Gorman, D., *The Body Moveable* (Ampersand, Guelph, Ontario, 1981).

97. Kapandji, I. A., *Physiology of the Joints* (Churchill Livingstone, New York, 1971).

98. Helms, J. M., *Acupuncture Energetics: A Clinical Approach for Physicians* (Medical Acupuncture Publishers, Berkeley, Ca., 1995).

99. Bucci, L., *Nutrition Applied to Injury Rehabilitation and Sports Injury* (CRC Press, Boca Raton, 1995).

100. Andrews, J. R., Harrelson, G. L., and Wilk, K., *Physical Rehabilitation of the Injured Athlete* (Saunders, Philadelphia, 1998).

101. Borgens, R., ed. *Electrical Fields in Vertebrate Repair* (Allen Liss, New York, 1989).

Bibliography

Abercrombie, M. and Dunn, G. A., "Locomotion and Contraction in Nonmuscle Cells," *Contractile Systems in Nonmuscle Tissues*, Perry S. V. and Margreth, A., eds. (Elsevier, Amsterdam, 1976).

Adams, L. M., "The Anatomy of Joints Related to Function," *Mechanics of Human Joints*, Radin, E. L. and Wright, V., eds. (Dekker, New York, 1990).

Akeson, W. H. and Frank, C. B., "Ligament Biology and Biomechanics," *AAOS Symposium on Sports Medicine: The Knee*, (Mosby, St. Louis 1985).

Austin M., *Acupuncture Therapy* (ASI Publishers, New York, 1972).

Barral, J. P., *Visceral Manipulation I and II* (Eastland, Seattle, 1987, 1989).

Barral, J. P., *The Thorax* (Eastland, Seattle, 1989).

Barral, J. P., *Urogenital Manipulation* (Eastland, Seattle, 1993).

Barral, J. P., *Manual Thermal Diagnosis* (Eastland,Seattle, 1996).

Basmajian, J. V. and DeLuca, C., *Muscles Alive* (Williams and Wilkins, Baltimore, 1985).

Becker, F., "The Meaning of Fascia and Fascial Continuity," *Osteopathic Annals*, 35–47 (June, 1975).

Becker, R. L. and Selden, G., *The Body Electric* (Dekker, New York, 1990).

Becker, R. L., *Cross Currents* (Putnam, New York, 1983).

Becker, R. L., "Electromagnetism and Life," *Modern Bioelectricity*, Marino, A.A., ed. (Dekker, New York, 1988).

Becker, Rol., "Diagnostic Touch I and II," *Yearbooks, Academy of Applied Osteopathy* (1963 and 1964).

Bogduk, N., "The Innervation of the Lumbar Spine," *Spine*, 8: 286–293 (1989).

Borgens, R., ed., *Electrical Fields in Vertebrate Repair* (Allen Liss, New York, 1989).

Bowling, R. and Rockar, P., "The Elbow Complex," *Orthopedic and Sports Physical Therapy*, Gould, J. and Davies, G., eds. (Mosby, St. Louis, 1985).

Butler, D., *Mobilization of the Nervous System* (Churchill Livingstone, Melbourne, 1991).

Butler, D. L., "Anterior Cruciate Ligament: Its Normal Response and Replacement," J. Orthop Res 7: 910–921 (1989).

Cailliet, R., *Soft Tissue Pain and Disability* (F.A. Davis, Philadelphia, 1996).

Cohen, B. B., Manuals for Courses in Body-Mind Centering (School for Body-Mind Centering, Amherst, Mass., 1977–1987).

Cohen, B. B., *Sensing, Feeling and Action* (Contact Editions, Northampton, Mass, 1993).

Currier, D. P. and Nelson, R. M., *Dynamics of Human Biological Tissue* (Davis, F.A., Philadelphia, 1992).

Cyriax, J., *Textbook of Orthopedic Medicine* (Bailliere Tindall, London, 1980).

Dvorak, J. and Dvorak, V., *Manual Medicine* (Verlag, New York, 1990).

Elzinga, M. and Lu, R., "Comparative Amino Acid Sequence Studies on Actin," *Contractile Systems in Nonmuscle Tissues*, Perry, S.V. and Margreth, A., eds. (Elsevier, Amsterdam, 1976).

Farfan, H., *Mechanical Disorders of the Low Back* (Lea and Febiger, Philadelphia, 1973).

Frankel, V. and Nordin, M., *Basic Biomechanics of the Skeletal System* (Lea and Febiger, Philadelphia, 1980).

Fryette, H. H., *Principles of Osteopathic Technic* (Acad. of Applied Osteopathy, California, 1954).

Frymann, V. M., "A Study of the Rhythmic Motions of the Living Cranium," *J. Am. Osteopath Association*, 70: 928–45 (1971).

Ganong, W., *Medical Physiology* (Appleton and Lange, Norwalk, Conn., 1992).

Garrick, J. and Radetsky, P., *Peak Fitness* (Crown, New York, 1986).

Gehin, A., *Atlas of Manipulative Techniques for the Cranium and Face* (Eastland Press, Seattle, 1985).

Gerber, R., *Vibrational Medicine* (Bear and Co., Santa Fe, 1988).

Gorman, D., *The Body Moveable* (Ampersand, Guelph, Ontario, 1981).

Gould, J. and Davies, G., eds., *Orthopedic and Sports Physical Therapy* (Mosby, St. Louis, 1985).

Grieve, G. P., ed., *Modern Manual Therapy of the Vertebral Column* (Churchill Livingstone, Edinburgh, 1986).

Guyton, A., *Textbook of Medical Physiology* (W.B. Saunders, Philadelphia, 1981).

Hoppenfeld, S., *Physical Examination of the Spine and Extremities* (Appleton-Century, Norwalk, Conn., 1976).

Hunt, T. K., Heppenstall, R. B., Pines E., eds., *Soft and Hard Tissue Repair* (Praeger, New York, 1980).

Hunt, V., *Infinite Mind: The Science of Human Vibrations* (Malibu, Malibu, Ca., 1995).

Johansson, H. and Sjolander, P., "Neurophysiology of Joints," *Mechanics of Human Joints*, Radin E.L. and Wright, V., eds. (Dekker, New York, 1990).

Jones, L. H., "Spontaneous Release by Positioning," DO 4: 109–16 (1964).

Jones, L. H., *Jones Strain-Counterstrain* (Jones Strain-Counterstrain Inc., Boise, Id. 1995).

Juhan, D., *Job's Body* (Station Hill Press, Barrytown, New York, 1987).

Kapandji, I. A., *Physiology of the Joints* (Churchill Livingstone, New York, 1971).

Kessler, R. and Hertling, D., eds., *Management of Common Musculoskeletal Disorders* (Lippincott, Philadelphia, 1990).

Kirkaldy-Willis, W., *Managing Low Back Pain* (Churchill Livingstone, New York, 1990).

Korr, I. M., *Collected Papers of I. M. Korr* (Amer. Acad. of Osteopathy, Colorado Springs, 1979).

Korr, I. M., ed., *Neurobiologic Mechanisms in Manipulative Therapy* (Plenum, New York, 1978).

Korr, I. M., "Neurochemical and Neurotrophic Consequences of Nerve Deformation," *Aspects of Manipulative Therapy*, Glasgow, E. F. Twomey, L.T., eds. (Churchill Livingstone, Edinburgh, 1985).

Lackie, J. M., ed., *Cell Movement and Cell Behavior* (Allen and Unwin, London, 1986).

Lehmkuhl, L. D. and Smith, L. K., *Brunnstrom's Clinical Kinesiology* (F. A. Davis, Philadelphia, 1983).

LeVeau, B. F., "Basic Biomechanics in Sports and Orthopedic Physical Therapy," *Orthopedic and Sports Physical Therapy*, Gould, J. and Davies, G., eds. (Mosby, St. Louis, 1985).

Lippincott, H. and R., *Manual of Cranial Technique* (Edwards Brothers, Ann Arbor, 1943).

Lundborg, G., *Nerve Injury and Repair* (Churchill Livingstone, Edinburgh, 1988).

Magoun, H. I., *Osteopathy in the Cranial Field* (Journal Printing, Kirksville, Mo., 1966).

Marino, A., ed., *Modern Bioelectricity*, (Dekker, New York, 1988).

Mauro, A., ed., *Muscle Regeneration* (Raven, New York, 1979).

McCarty, D. J. and Koopman, W. J., eds., *Arthritis and Allied Conditions: A Textbook of Rheumatology* (Lea and Febiger, Philadelphia, 1993).

McConaill, M. A. and Basmajian, J. V., *Muscles and Movements* (Krieger, New York, 1977).

McPartland, J. M. and Mein, E. A., "Entrainment and the Cranial Rhythmic Impulse," *J. Alternative Therapies in Health and Medicine*, 1: 40–46 (1997).

Melzack, R. and Wall, P., *Textbook of Pain* (Churchill Livingstone, Edinburgh, 1984).

Mow, V., Ratcliffe, A., Savio, L., eds., *Biomechanics of Diarthrodial Joints* (Springer-Verlag, New York, 1990).

Murphy, M., *Future of the Body* (Tarcher, Los Angeles, 1992).

Nachmias, D. and Nachmias, C., *Research Methods* (Plenum, New York, 1987).

Norkin, C. and Levangie, P., *Joint Structure and Function* (F.A. Davis, Philadelphia, 1992).

Noyes, F. R., DeLucas, J. L., "Biomechanics of Anterior Cruciate Ligament Failure," *J. Bone and Joint Surgery*, 56: 236–253 (1974).

Palastanga, N., "Transverse Friction Massage," *Modern Manual Therapy of the Vertebral Column*, Grieve, G.P., ed. (Churchill Livingstone, Edinburgh, 1986).

Patton, M. Q., *Qualitative Evaluation and Research Methods* (Sage, Newbury Park, Ca., 1990).

Perry, S.V. and Margreth, A., eds., *Contractile Systems in Nonmuscle Tissues* (Elsevier, Amsterdam, 1976).

Pollard, T. and Fujiwara, K., eds., "Participation of Contractile Proteins in Cytoplasmic Stractive and Cell Division," *Contractile Systems in Nonmuscle Tissues*, Perry, S. V. and Margreth, A., eds. (Elsevier, Amsterdam, 1976).

Radin, E. L. and Wright, V., eds., *Mechanics of Human Joints* (Dekker, New York, 1990).

Radin, E. L., "Osteoarthritis," *Mechanics of Human Joints*, Radin, E. L. and Wright, V., eds. (Dekker, New York, 1990).

Reichmanis, M., "Electro-acupuncture," *Modern Bioelectricity*, Marino, A. A., ed. (Dekker, New York, 1988).

Retzlaff, E. W. and Mitchell, F. L., eds., *The Cranium and its Sutures* (Springer-Verlag, New York, 1987).

Rolf, I. P., *Rolfing: The Integration of Human Structures* (Harper and Row, 1977).

Simkin, P. A., "Biology of Joints," *Mechanics of Human Joints*, Radin, E. L. and Wright, V., eds. (Dekker, New York, 1990).

Sisken, B., "Effects of Electromagnetic Fields on Nerve Regeneration," *Modern Bioelectricity*, Marino, A. A., ed. (Dekker, New York, 1988).

Skalak, R. and Chien, S., *Handbook of Bioengineering* (Springer-Verlag, New York, 1987).

Smith, F. F., *Inner Bridges* (Humanics, Atlanta, 1990).

Smith, S., "Limb Regeneration," *Modern Bioelectricity*, Marino, A. A., ed. (Dekker, New York, 1990).

Stoddard, A., *Manual of Osteopathic Technique* (Hutchison, London, 1980).

Strohman, R., Yamada, S., Buffinger, N., "Fibroblast Growth Factor Plays a Role in Regulating Muscle Hypertrophy," *Medicine and Science in Sports and Exercise*, Am. Coll. of Sports Medicine: S 173–80 (1989).

Studitskii, A. N., *Transplantation of Muscles in Animals* (Oxonian, New Delhi, 1988).

Subotnick, S. and Sisney, P., "Treatment of Achilles Tendinopathy in the Athlete," *J. Am. Podiatric Medical Association.*, 76: 10, 552–556 (1987).

Sutherland, W. G., *The Cranial Bowl* (Free Press, Mankato, Minn., 1939).

Sutherland, W. G., Sutherland, A. S., Wales, A., eds., *The Collected Writings of William Garner Sutherland* (Sutherland Cranial Teaching Foundation, Kansas City, 1967).

Todd, M. E., *The Thinking Body* (Dance Horizons, New York, 1936).

Viidik, A. and Gottrup, F., "Mechanics of Healing Soft Tissue Wounds," *Frontiers in Biomechanics*, Woo, S. L., Schmid-Schonbein, G. W., Zweifach, B. W., eds. (Springer-Verlag, New York, 1986).

Viidik, A. and Vuust, J., eds., *Biology of Collagen* (Academic Press, London, 1980).

Williamson, S. J., ed., *Biomagnetism: An Interdisciplinary Approach* (Plenum, New York, 1983).

Wyke, B. D., "Neurology of the Cervical Spinal Joints," *Physiotherapy*, 65: 72 (1979).

Wyke, B. D., "Articular Neurology and Manipulative Therapy," *Aspects of Manipulative Therapy*, Idczak, I. M., ed. (Lincoln Institute of Health Sciences, Victoria, Australia, 1980).

Wyke, B. D. and Polacek, P., "Articular Neurology: The Present Position," *J. Bone Joint Surgery* 57B (1975).

Yin, R. K., *Case Study Research* (Sage, Thousand Oaks, Ca., 1994).

Index

About the Author

William Weintraub has a Masters degree in Biomechanics from Antioch University. He has practiced and taught structural/osteopathic therapy in the San Francisco Bay Area for twenty-five years. He has trained extensively in osteopathic and related methods including Practitioner Certifications in Body-Mind Centering and acupressure therapy.